# THE PHAT CHICK

# THE PHAT CHICK

## NOW I EAT TO LIVE,
## AND DON'T LIVE TO EAT

## KELLI HARSHA

**To order additional copies of this book, contact:**
Xlibris Corporation
1-888-795-4274
www.Xlibris.com
Orders@Xlibris.com
56240

# Contents

# DEDICATION

First and foremost to my Lord and Savior, who has given me the ultimate strength to reach my goals. I know without a shadow of a doubt, that with you as my rock, I can never fail.

In memory of my grandmother, Alice Moore, who was the first person who ever made the comment "Man, are you big!". I know that it wasn't meant to be mean, it was just the truth! But sometimes we need to hear the truth to make the change that will last forever. I love you and miss you with all my heart. Till we meet again.

To my beloved mother, Phyllis, thank you for all the times you just lent an ear, a hug, or a hand in prayer. You have given me strength, support, and the courage to stand for what I believe; and I love you so much. To my Father, Kenny. Thank you for being an important part of my life. I love you, Dad.

To my children, Kaytlyn Elizabeth and little Jerry. God blessed my life with the birth of my two angels. You are both precious gifts from heaven and I love you so much. My best friend, Bo Bo, without love and support from home, none of this would be possible. I thank you for encouraging me to strive for my dreams, and my goals. You and Taylor have taken a special place in my heart, and I love you both dearly.

# PREFACE

Today is the first day of the rest of your life. That is a phrase that many have heard and even have said. The thought has passed through many minds and traveled through many mouths. I never really paid any attention to what that meant until I ultimately made the decision to change my life and my own thought process. I was very overweight after the birth of my second child and, little to my dismay, was even at a place in my life that I didn't even care. I was married with two children and living my life for my kids and my husband in my own comfort zone, which is what most women in their twenties try to achieve. At least I thought I was in my comfort zone. Now, I know that I was in everyone else's comfort zone, and I was just trailing along, blending. I wanted to make everyone happy. I always have tried to be a people pleaser, and you know there is nothing wrong with that. But it is so easy to literally lose who you are and what your purpose is in life. Are we here for others, or are we here for ourselves? The last year and a half, I have done a lot of learning about who I am. Soul searching, so to speak. I want to leave this earth one day knowing that I did everything that I could have done to change people's lives. There is no greater strength than that of an individual who overcomes whatever obstacles may arise in their life. My hope and my dream for each person that may pick up this book is that they will realize where they truly are in their life and know that we only have today. Don't put off till tomorrow what you may achieve today. With Great Sacrifice Comes Great Reward. Whether you struggle with weight loss or just insecurities within yourself, nothing can be changed or altered, unless you fix it from the inside out. No matter what your individual goals may be, IF YOU CAN SEE IT AND YOU BELIEVE IT, THEN YOU CAN ACHIEVE IT AND BE IT!

God bless you.

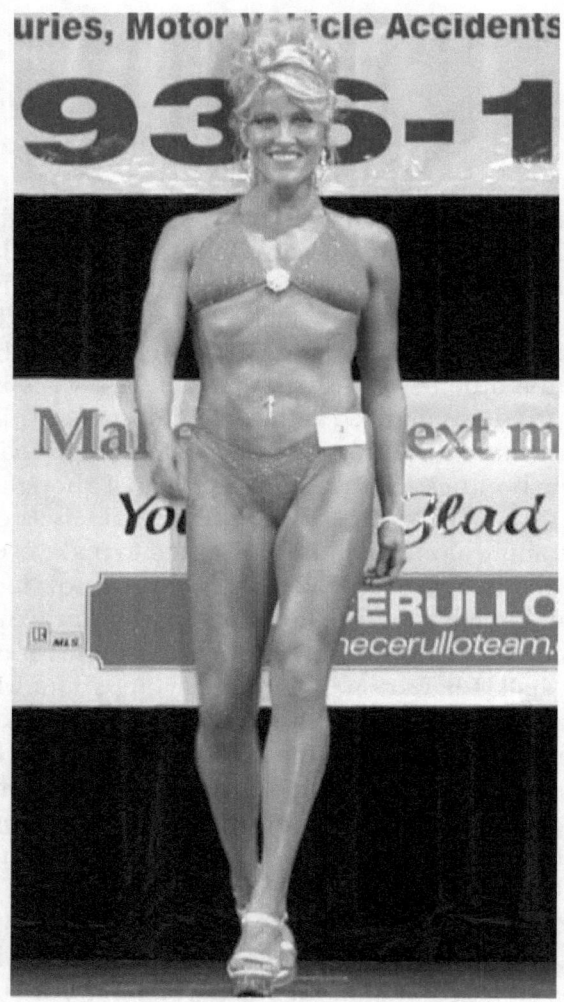

# HOW COME THEY GOT IT AND I DON'T?

Have you ever been to a gym or fitness center and witnessed the woman with the perfect body? The type of body that just can't be for real because we all know that no one ever looks that good! Or the guy with muscles protruding from every part of his body, including the veins and the muscular striations that we all just look at in utter amazement at how could anybody honestly get their body to look like that? Let's face it people, IT'S NOT FAIR! That's how it seems anyway, doesn't it? I remember trying to find an outfit to work out in, something that would make me appear a little smaller than what I was (which was hard at two hundred and some-odd pounds), only to find a baggy pair of sweat pants and an oversized T-shirt that I would hide under, to drag my fat butt to the gym to spend ungodly hours on a boring cardio machine while I would watch the hard bodies and skinny little rear ends walking by. Gasping for air as I watched every second ticking away, hoping that one day that would be my skinny little rear end walking through the gym! Little did I know, at the time, that most of those people not only had to work very hard for what they had, but that hard work also continued in just maintaining that kind of physique. I knew in my heart of hearts that despite what I saw in the mirror every day, I was a long-lost fitness chick, with a great body stuck behind the fat and blubber of a modern day woman. I didn't know how to get there or where to start, but I knew that I had reached a point in my life that I needed to make a change.

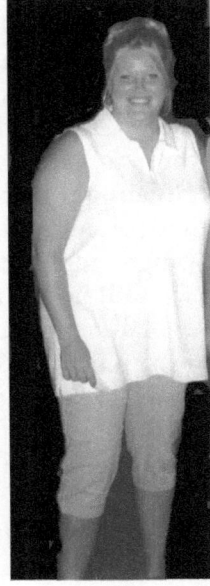

It's funny how when you are heavy and overweight, it is so easy to put on a happy mask and pretend that you are so satisfied with who you are. Even if you honestly just don't feel that well, physically or mentally. I believe that some people that are overweight, are happy. Their self-confidence is unbelievable. They are at peace with who they are and what they look like. I, my friends, was not one of them. I was tired of being fat. I was tired of going shopping for clothes and buying one of the biggest sizes on the rack. I was tired of being tired and having no energy and, in all honesty, not even really caring that I had no energy. Unless you have been in that position, you wouldn't even know what I am talking about; but if you have been or if you currently are, let me just say from my experience, life is so much better when you can actually live it to the fullest and overcome those personal obstacles.

Throughout my journey, over the last few years, one question that everyone always asks me is "What made you decide to start losing weight? Was there a moment or a turning point?" The answer, my friend, is that I ultimately was just tired of the way I felt physically and emotionally; and I hated the way that I looked. My self-esteem was so low that words cannot express how I felt when I looked in the mirror. I guess when you hit that point, you can only keep going and get worse, or you can honestly put things into perspective and make a change that will eventually change your life for the better, forever.

I am here to help you and to encourage you that you can do it. You can make the change that will not only make you feel better about yourself, but you can make a change that you know in your heart will add years to your life. In the chapters to follow, I am going to give you not only advice and tips to keep you on track, but I will also add in some recipes and pointers that will help keep you motivated. Remember, great change doesn't occur overnight; it takes time. Just as it took time for you to get to where you are today, it will take time to get you where you need to be and to maintain that for the rest of your life. I can tell you from experience that you are going to have days and probably even weeks that you are going to fall off the bandwagon and want to give up. But please, for your own well being, don't. Don't ever give up on your dreams or your goals, no matter what they may be.

You have taken the first step, so don't let another Monday go by. We all say "Okay that's it. Starting Monday, I am starting my diet!" How about starting on a Tuesday or Wednesday just for kicks, and don't look at this journey as a DIET! Look at it as you are making a significant change in your life, for the rest of your life, and your brand-new nutritional way of life journey begins today.

# YOUR NEW BEGINNING

So you have decided to make a change. Whether you need to add on some lean muscle, just tone up, or shed some unwanted pounds, you have now made a decision that most people may never make. To get healthier means far more than just changing a few things in your diet. It is a complete lifestyle change, and it too can even help your family and loved ones become more aware of their physical and personal habits. Whether you are making a change for yourself, helping a spouse, a loved one, or a child, we will discuss some of the main tools that you are going to need to get moving in the right direction.

First and foremost, your diet is EVERYTHING. Hear me say it again. Nutrition is EVERYTHING! I don't care how much you are at the gym, how many thousands of miles you have rode on a bike, walked on a treadmill, or rowed on a machine. If your diet isn't in line, then you are wasting time with all the exercise. Don't take this wrong. I mean exercise is wonderful for your heart and your muscles, cardio and strength, but if you are trying to make a distinct and definite change in your health and your physique, your eating habits are 80 percent of your change. You can make a significant change in your body by just changing the way that you eat. Have you ever heard anyone say "Man, I've stopped drinking pop, and you know I've lost ten pounds." There you have it. That is a prime example of how a small change in your nutritional habits alone can alter a change physically.

Look at it like this. How many times have you been to the gym and have noticed the same people that have been there every day, all the time, and their physique hasn't changed at all? Pay attention because I'll tell you what, you can work out until you are blue in the face, but if your diet isn't clean, your workouts are pretty much worthless. I know each and every one of you, when you are doing your cardio, watch that machine tick away at how many calories you have burned. It seems like it takes forever to burn a significant amount, and what good does it do to work out so hard and leave the gym to run through fast-food and take in more calories than you just burned off? The same is true, however, if you never walked or exercised a day in your life, but decided to change your eating habits, you would lose weight. Unfortunately, you'd lose some lean body mass along with body fat.

The idea when you are beginning to alter your body composition is to keep lean muscle and add to it. Muscle burns fat. That's it, plain and simple. If your diet is clean and you are doing cardio and some resistance training, then your long-term goals will so be reached.

When I say your "diet," I am referring to your nutritional way of life. No one likes to be on a diet. Let's face it, it is the dreaded word, and if you are going on a diet, you are probably going to go off your diet. You need to find a new nutritional way of life. A persistent way to live your life normally is not depriving yourself or your family of the things that you love. My best advice to my clients is to allow one cheat meal a week, but make sure that it is consistent with the same time every week. Don't have a cheat meal on a Saturday one week and then decide that Monday you are going to have your cheat meal for that week. When I refer to a "cheat" meal, I mean whatever you can consume in one sitting: appetizer, drink, dinner, and dessert. Eat your heart out for one meal a week, but only one. Remember you are the one that has to be accountable for your actions. If you are honest with yourself and you only have one cheat meal a week that you really allow yourself to splurge, you are not going to damage your weight-loss goal from one meal. However, if you are training for a bodybuilding or figure competition, my advice would be a bit different. Right now, I am talking about your basic nutrition, and when you are starting a great change in your eating habits, it will be easier for you to be consistent on your nutritional way of life, when you allow yourself that one free meal. Is it really going to be feasible for you or your family to eat clean 100 percent of the time? Nope, be reasonable, and do allow yourself an occasional splurge!

So now you need to figure out what your goal is. Do you want to lose unwanted pounds or add on muscle mass or both? Are you trying to transform yourself or your entire family? It is very important that you remember your children will most likely pick up your habits. If you eat badly, so will your children. If you are faithful with eating right and exercising, your children will most likely follow in your footsteps. Some words of advice to follow:

1.  STAY OFF THE SCALE. I would say, as women, we always know what we weigh, and what we would love to weigh. Men, I'm not sure if they care what the scale says as much as what the tape measure says when it's wrapped around their bicep! The fact of

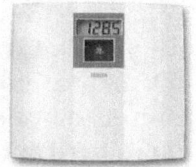

the matter is that the number on the scale honestly doesn't matter. Your consistency with body fat percentage loss and lean body mass gain are two very important key factors with getting the physique that you're wanting. First of all, if you are doing any kind of resistance training or strength training (which we'll get into more later in the book), you need to learn that muscle weighs more than fat; so if you are lifting weights or using resistance bands in your training, you ARE going to put on lean muscle, which is why you may not notice a significant change in the scale at first. Not only does muscle weigh more than fat, but it also takes up less space. Look at it like this: a person that is in a size 24 jeans could weigh the same as a person in a size 16 jeans, being that the size 16 has more lean mass than the size 24.

Another very important note is muscle burns fat; therefore, the more muscle or lean body mass that you have, the more susceptible your body is to burning fat. With my clients, I will only use the scale to figure out body fat pounds and lean body mass pounds. I don't believe for one second that anyone should base their total weight loss on the scale. People don't realize how important your body fat and lean mass really are. You should always go by your clothes. How are they fitting? Try using a piece of clothing to judge your inches lost, rather than using the scale with pounds lost. Today's society has become so obsessed with what the scale says, when in reality, it has overcome so many aspects of our daily lives. I know people that will get up first thing every morning and weigh themselves. What good does that do? I know from my experience after I hit 250 lbs. I did NOT want to get on that scale! You couldn't have forced me to get on it! Weighing yourself constantly is going to do nothing but set yourself up for disappointment. Your body is going to change, but it is not going to happen overnight. It didn't happen overnight for me, and I'm telling you, it won't happen overnight for you either. But the good news is that it can happen, and it will. I promise.

2.   EAT OFTEN AND EAT SMALL AMOUNTS. You have probably heard this many times and perhaps never really understood why. Well, this is why. When you get up in the morning and eat your breakfast, your belly is full, and you feel great (depending on what you ate for your breakfast). Let's just say that 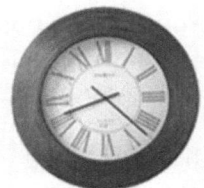 the day gets going, and you are so busy that you don't have time to eat. Before you know it, it's dinnertime, and you are so hungry you could eat your arm; so you eat whatever you can get your hands on, then before you know it, you are so stuffed you can't move. When you

eat breakfast in the morning, you have just started your metabolism going, so you sent it into express mode; however, when you chose not to eat or you get so busy that you don't make time, your body begins to think that you are not feeding it, therefore, sending it into a "resting metabolic state." Basically what this means is that when you don't eat, your body actually thinks that you are not going to feed it; so when you finally decide to consume some food, it keeps it, thus, storing most of it as fat solely because it isn't sure when you are going to feed it again.

Now, take the same example, but let's change it up a bit. You get up in the morning and decide that you are going to do some cardio, whether a nice brisk walk or morning jog, before you ever put anything in your stomach. After about thirty minutes of cardio, you eat some breakfast. You then decide to plan your day of meals and prepare that you are going to eat something with some nutritional value in it about every three to four hours all day long and just before you go to bed. Yes, that's right! Eat a high protein, low-fat meal or drink a high protein drink and go straight to bed. It's very hard to eat six times a day, so I recommend eating three meals and drinking three high protein shakes a day. The first thing that you are going to notice is that you will most likely not be hungry when it is time for you to eat again, but you must eat. Do not let your body get hungry like it did in our last example. The next thing you may notice is that you probably won't get tired in the afternoon.

Most people crash mid-afternoon because with their lunch, they probably didn't eat the right combination of foods, and their afternoon snack is most likely not really what we would call a healthy snack. However, because you have now planned out your day and you are prepared, you now get home from work. Its dinner time, and what do you know? Your arm is still there! What has happened is that you have sparked a "kick" in your metabolism from the time you got out of bed. You did your cardio on an empty stomach, which will make your body have to tap into your stored body fat for energy, so your metabolism has turned into a fat-burning machine. You then eat after you do your cardio, so now not only is your metabolism moving; but when you eat, believe it or not, you are keeping your body fat burning. The idea of eating every three to four hours is going to keep your body in a fat-burning state. You want to keep your metabolism going all day, so you don't want to get to that point that you are so hungry that you are ready to eat your arm or your leg! The best way to do this is keep eating consistently all day every three to four hours. And to do that you HAVE to prepare and plan out what you are going to eat and when you are going to eat it.

The same is true for your kids. How many times have you sent your child to school, and they are racing out the door, pop tart in hand. Probably more times than not. We have to teach our children that we don't just say that "breakfast is the most important meal of the day." It really and truly is. Make sure that your child has a snack to have at least mid-afternoon to keep them from experiencing that crash too. The same scenario works with our children. We are living in a fast-food frenzy world, my friends, and our children are on the verge of being the wounded victims because we are not teaching them how to live a full, complete, healthy life. It is our job as parents, teachers, aunts, and uncles to embrace our children and help lead them into a better direction of healthy living.

3. DRINK LOTS OF WATER. The more water you drink, the better. I know that you have ALL heard this one before, but believe it or not, if you do not drink enough water, you could get fatter. Bet you never thought you'd here that one, but it is true. When you drink water, it helps your liver effectively metabolize body fat. Not drinking enough water can cause glucose to be stored as fat. "Okay," you 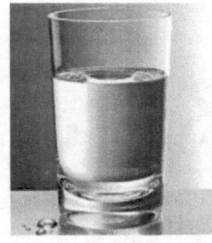 say, "what exactly is glucose?" Well, the dictionary basically defines glucose as a monosaccharide (or simple sugar) also known as grape sugar. It is an important carbohydrate in biology. The living cell uses it as a source of energy and metabolic function. So basically not drinking enough water means that you're not utilizing your body to complete its function. You are not flushing your system of toxins, and sodium or feeding your organs to function right. A lot of people say that they just can't drink water and they have a hard time consuming it. Try adding some green tea or flavored drink packets to your water, and you would be surprised how much that will help. On the same note, our families need the direction steered away from the fountain and soda drinks and focused more on $H_2O$. Our bodies are made up of 50 to 60 percent fluids, so we need to continuously replenish our fluids with water.

4. PERFORM CARDIO AT EITHER A LOWER INTENSITY OR IN INTERVALS. When you perform your cardio or aerobic activity at a lower intensity, rather than high, it will promote a greater loss of body fat. Your body prefers to use stored body fat for energy rather than carbohydrates for fuel. If 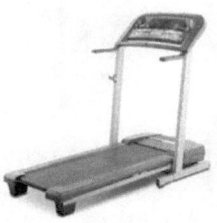 you interval circuit train, you allow your heart rate to escalate and then decrease, therefore, not letting your heart rate race

for a long period of time and again allowing your body to utilize stored fat for energy rather than burning carbohydrates. Try to keep your heart rate in fat-burning range (220 – [your age] x .65) for the low end of your fat burning heart rate, and (220 – [your age] x .85) for the high end of your fat burning heart rate. Keeping your heart rate in the range of these two numbers will increase your fat burning mode. Remember too, that the best time to do your cardio is in the morning on an empty stomach before you eat anything. The reason for this is because when you wake up, your glycogen stores or sugars are low and, thus, can be depleted quickly, causing your body to have no choice but to use its stored fat for energy rather than the extra calories acquired from an early meal.

5.  CONSUME FIBER. Fiber is a very important nutritional key factor in your nutritional daily life. Fiber is filling without fattening. It stays in the stomach longer; so it absorbs water, swells, and helps the eater 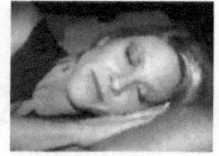 feel full. Consuming fifteen to twenty-five grams of fiber a day will not only "keep you regular," but it slows fat absorption. It also helps lower your cholesterol, steadies your blood sugar level, reduces cancer risks, and promotes healthy intestinal bacteria. Good sources of Fiber, include 100% bran cereal, raisins, prunes, fruit, beans, broccoli, and green veggies.

6.  SLEEP. Your body does most of its recovery and growing at night when you are sleeping. Not when you're in the gym, burning out the muscle, or walking on the treadmill. Yes, as soon as you are done with your workout, your body is starting to recover; however, it is when you are allowing your body to rest at night when you are truly recovering. It is imperitive that you try to get at least 8 hours of sleep at night. Muscles need rest and protein to grow; it's a basic fact. Since your muscles are going to grow and recover while you are sleeping, why not feed your muscles some protein. I recommend 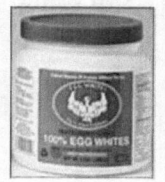 a pure liquid egg white protein shake right before you hit the pillow. **YUK!** Yes, that's the first thing I said too. **YUK!** However, I found the most amazing 100 percent pure liquid egg whites by a company called Egg Whites International. They are pasteurized and *Salmonella* safe. And best of all, they are not slimy. They double filter them to remove all the slimy texture, so they are smooth like milk. That means no slimy taste. Liquid egg whites are a time-release protein, so they support muscle and work in your body for up to four to five hours or most of your sleep time. The best protein powders on the

market today are only 70 to 80 percent bio-available for only two to three hours of muscle support. For those of you that don't know what bio-available means, basically, if you use twenty grams of a protein powder, your body can only breakdown and use about 70 percent or fourteen grams of the twenty grams supplied by the powder. One hundred percent Pure Liquid Egg Whites will use 100 percent of the protein. By consuming the liquid egg whites, you are going to feed your body all night long. Rather than eating a carbohydrate that is going to lie in your belly and eventually turn into fat because the chances of you getting up at two o'clock in the morning and doing some cardio are probably slim to none!

7.   PLAN, PREPARE, AND BE ACCOUNTABLE. Probably the best advice that I can give you is perhaps one that you honestly probably already know. If you do not plan and you do not prepare ahead of time, you will not be successful. 'Failing to Plan, is Planning to Fail.' You have to be ready every day, every meal, for what you are going to do. When we do not prepare, we give in to cravings and easy access to food that we know we shouldn't be consuming. Don't get me wrong. We are all human, and there is no better joy than just going on an eating binge, consuming all the things that we love. What perhaps you don't realize is once you start being accountable for what and how much you are eating, when you do cheat or splurge, you will find that you honesty won't feel that great. You'll be bloated and uncomfortable afterward. It's great to let loose and just eat what we want every once in a while, but sometimes old habits are hard to break, and it is so easy to go back to how things used to be. So be careful. There is no greater honesty within ourselves than when we have to be accountable for what we eat and how much we exercise.

Before you actually start your brand-new nutritional way of living, keep track for three days everything that you eat. After you write down those first three days, add up your calories. You will be surprised by either how much, or how little, you actually ate. Then when you start really being accountable of your new change, you will notice how much your old habits are going be hard to break. No matter what, you need to write down everything. Basically, if it goes in your mouth, it goes in your journal. You should never eat anything without writing it down. You have to keep track of what you are consuming so you know when detailed changes need to be made in your diet. When you finally reach your goal, you will be maintaining; and by then, your entire nutritional way of life will be different, and you will just automatically know what you should and shouldn't eat and when.

People don't realize that when you "graze" throughout the day, you are actually taking in so many more calories than you'd ever think. Journaling is a great way to be accountable. It really helps put into perspective what you are putting in your mouth. Just as you journal for your nutrition, though, you should also journal with your exercise program. You need to keep track of what body part you are working out, how many reps and sets, and how much cardio you are doing. I know you are thinking, my gosh, what a pain in the butt. Yeah, but look at it like this, 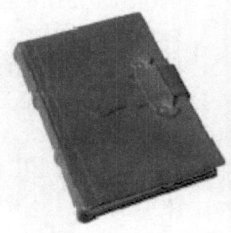 how bad do you want a change? It has to come from within yourself; and if you are not ready, none of my advice, or anyone else's for that matter, is going to make a difference in your life. You are the only one that can change your habits.

# OUT WITH THE OLD, IN WITH THE NEW

Like I had mentioned in the last chapter, you have to want a change more than anything in your life. There are so many factors within our daily life such as school, career, families, and friends that we let take over our nutritional and fitness decisions. Have you ever really stopped to realize that everything that we do pretty much revolves around food? That is why so many people say, "Well, I'm just going to start a diet on Monday." Monday never comes, and why? Everything in our lives from company meetings, family time, holidays, and luncheons revolves around food. So that is where the new you comes into play. You have to start making new healthier decisions within your lifestyle. Running to baseball practices, ballerina recitals, piano lessons, and football games and still utilize the "healthier eating" thinking game. "Okay," you say, "so how do I know what to eat, when to eat it, and how much to eat?" Well, I thought that you would never ask!

The first step is to figure out how much you weigh, your body fat, and your lean body mass. This can be done at a local fitness center or your family physician, a nutritionist, or a personal trainer. Not hard to find. Keep track of your daily caloric intake by journaling. You must write down everything. This is how you are going to know when you will need to adjust your daily caloric intake as pounds are lost and lean muscle is gained. So to lose weight you should calculate your total calories that you need to consume by taking your desired weight and multiplying it by 10 if you are a woman, and by 11, if you are a man. So if you are a female and your current weight is 200 pounds and you are wanting to weigh 150 pounds, you should eat a 1500-calorie diet. If you are a 350-pound man and you're wanting to weigh 170 pounds, you should take in 1870 calories a day. Remember, though, when you are doing resistance training and cardio, which you absolutely should do, YOU HAVE TO EAT! A lot of people are mistaken by the idea that if they workout or do some cardio, they are going to lose more weight if they don't eat. WRONG! Again, remember this, the more you exercise, the more HEALTHIER eating that you need to do. Eat every three to four hours and eat right. If you don't feed your body, you may allow yourself to fall into that resting metabolic state or a starvation mode. You could potentially lose little body fat, causing your body to tap into lean muscle for energy. You actually may trick your body into starvation mode, where it will think that you are depriving it. Unfortunately, what that means is that when you do eventually eat, your body will store it, thinking that you're not going to feed it again—not soon enough anyway.

At first when you are just trying to lose weight, I definitely suggest that you watch your calories. Burning more calories than you consume is going to help you burn fat; but remember, if you are not doing resistance training, you will probably lose some lean muscle too. The trick is to keep as much lean muscle as you can and lose as much body fat as you can. Don't forget the more lean muscle that you have, the more your body will continue to burn fat when you are not in exercise mode.

Muscle burns fat. One of the best ways to constantly feed your muscles is with liquid egg whites. Not raw egg whites, liquid egg whites. **What's the difference?** The human body cannot completely and safely digest a raw egg white. So if you like to do the "Rocky Routine" with a raw egg or raw egg white in your drink, you are wasting your time, not to mention the threat of *Salmonella*. Avidin, which is found in raw egg whites, blocks the uptake of Vitamin B6 (Biotin), causing a vitamin deficiency. You must cook the egg white to neutralize the Avidin and allow your body to safely digest the protein and utilize all its amino acids. Unfortunately, cooking also starts to destroy the protein. You lose about 12 percent of the protein when you cook the egg white.

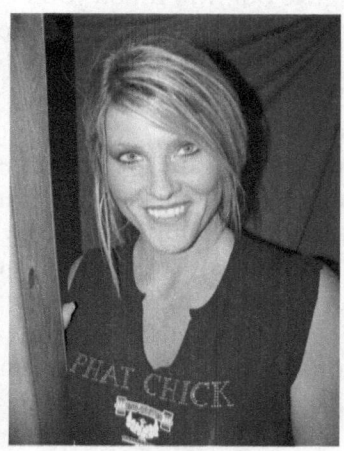

As I mentioned earlier, the 100 percent pure liquid egg whites from **Egg Whites International** are heat pasteurized and *Salmonella* tested. The pasteurization process heats the egg white to 134 degrees for 3½ minutes. This heat kills the *Salmonella* and neutralizes the Avidin to allow the egg whites to be digested safely by the human body. When you cook an egg white to the point of scrambled eggs, you are overcooking the protein and denaturing the true value of the protein. Therefore, 100 percent Pure Liquid Egg Whites are liquid, but not raw, making them the purest form of protein **in the entire world!** They make great omelets, but they are better for you as a drink, and it is the most beneficial way of bringing in that significant source of protein into your diet. Anyone can drink them, and everyone will benefit from them.

**How much protein should you get a day?** The average active person should consume about one gram of protein per pound of lean body weight per day. So if your lean body weight is 120 pounds, but you weigh 180 pounds, you should take in 120 grams of protein per day. Calculate from your lean weight, not your actual weight. So take 120 grams divided by at least five meals a day, and you need 24 grams of protein per meal. This calculation will help you maintain the lean muscle mass that you already have, and help you build a little bit more. Remember this, there are 4 calories per 1 gram of protein.

However, if you are wanting to add on more muscle mass, as in a Bodybuilding or Figure competition diet, you should consume one and a half grams of protein per pound of lean body weight per day. This will definitely help you add on a more significant amount of lean muscle. The same calculation is true as in the previous paragraph, so if your lean body weight is 120 pounds, you would multiply this by 1.5, getting you to 180 grams of protein per day, which would then be divided by at least 5 meals, giving you 36 grams of protein per meal.

Throughout this book, you will read about the benefits of liquid egg whites from Egg Whites International. They were very instrumental, as I was able to consume more protein in my meals, and know that my body was going to utilize ALL of the protein. When you eat any source of protein whether it is chicken, fish, steak, or tuna your body can only digest so much of the protein. Your stomach has to break down the food for your body to utilize the nutrients, causing you to not actually utilize all the protein that is in the food. Not to be gross, but when you eat a big protein meal like chicken, fish or steak, you are in the bathroom having a reading session within a few hours. However, when you drink the liquid egg whites, your body doesn't have to break down anything. It absorbs and uses everything because it is in liquid form, therefore, causing all the nutrients and protein found in the drink to be 100 percent used by the body. No reading session in the bathroom in a few hours. What an awesome way to get the daily protein intake into your nutritional needs. And it's very light on your stomach, unlike a heavy meal, which is why a lot of doctors, are actually recommending the liquid egg whites for gastric bypass patients. It is a beneficial way for patients of such surgeries to really be able to get in their protein intake.

Now, I am not a fan of the surgery nor will you ever hear me recommend it to anyone; and if you want my personal opinion, I think that it is a fast fix-it, with lessons going unlearned. We are all entitled to our own opinions. However, I have seen and heard of so many people that have gone through such surgeries and have either hit a plateau or have literally gotten sick, or put weight back on. Society today wants the quick fix. Yet no one wants to really work for it. It takes time. That's it. If you want a healthy, significant change in your life, it takes time. Yes, it's overwhelming, but what do you honestly learn by someone cutting your stomach in half or tying it off? You learn that you just can't eat the way that you used to. But that's because your body won't let you. Why not really teach yourself how to live a healthy life, instead of putting a rubber band around your stomach. That's only my opinion; take it with a grain of salt!

Moving on, so now you know how many calories you need to consume daily to lose weight, but that doesn't mean that you can just eat anything that you want. You have to eat healthy. Our bodies need protein, carbs, and fat. Yes, they need fat! I know that you are all thinking, "Well, I got enough of that for a lifetime!" Don't we all? The fact is that our bodies need good fats. "Good Fats?" you say, "are there really such a thing? Cuz all my fat is not good!"

Good fats that we can get from fish oil, omega-3, flaxseed oil, and olive oils—these are all great sources of good fats. Did you know that fat burns fat? Yes, indeed, it does. But the good fats, of course. There are 9 calories per 1 gram of fat. Dietary fats supply some of the best and most stable sources of energy. So if you want to feel better all day long, you need to make sure you are getting enough fats and the right types. The human body NEEDS fat just to function properly. Certain amounts of fat are necessary for proper hormone production. If your hormone production is off, so will your metabolism be, and you may not know this; but your hormones regulate many things in the body, including your ability to build and maintain muscle tissue, which is responsible for a great portion of your energy expenditure. To put it simply, your muscle mass will burn calories twenty-four hours a day, and if you eat a low-fat or no-fat diet, you will have a hard time building and maintaining muscle.

So listen, if you want to lose weight and be healthy, DON'T eat a low-fat diet. Eat a diet with healthy fat!

We talked about daily protein intake in the previous paragraph, so now we are going to touch base on carbs. We kind of discussed this in the previous chapter a bit. But how many carbs should you take in, and what kinds of carbs are good, and what kinds are bad? Well, let's begin. Remember, everyone needs carbs. Your body needs carbs for energy and to help feed your muscles. Fifty percent of your daily caloric intake should come from carbs. In order to find out how many carbs you should consume in a day, take the number of calories you need by .5. For example say you are on a 2,000 calorie diet. 2,000 calories multiplied by .5 equals 1,000. So 1,000 calories of your daily intake should come from carbohydrates. To figure how many grams of carbs are in the 1,000 calories . . . there are 4 calories in 1 gram of carbs. So take your 1,000 and divide by 4, will give you 250 grams of carbs, per day. This calculation may vary also depending on your activity level.

I don't care what books you have read, or what diets you have been on in the past. People today have been led to believe that carbohydrates are bad. CARBOHYDRATES ARE NOT BAD. Our bodies need them for energy. They are the major energy source for fuel in our bodies. Most people don't realize the effect that carbohydrates have on protein. They are known to "save the protein," meaning the carbs protect the protein that you consume from converting to glucose and being used for energy. When your carb intake is low, you have no energy. Your body has to find energy somewhere, so it goes within itself, tapping into lean muscle for its energy source. This puts you into pretty much a muscle wasting state.

Carbohydrates also serve in aiding in the proper developing and functioning of the central nervous system. The brain uses blood glucose for its main energy source—glucose as being found in the carbs that you digest. However, the brain does not store this glucose. It receives it from our daily nutrition, which now explains to you why the last time you were on a low-carb diet, your elevator most likely didn't go all the way to the top floor.

There are two types of carbs: complex carbs and simple carbs. The difference? A simple carb is a carbohydrate that your body will utilize and burn fast, such as fruit. A complex carb is going to be more your starches, sweet potatoes, baked potatoes, rice, pasta, oatmeal. A complex carb will stay in your body longer, giving you a longer-lasting feeling of being full, where a simple carb will burn up quickly and most the time cause your body to crash.

When you are doing resistance training, you are burning out the muscle. YOU WANT THE BURN! I have heard many people say that they don't like to hurt, or they don't like the burn. The fact of the matter is that if it ain't burnin', it ain't workin'! Why do you think they say "No Pain, No Gain?" Carbohydrates help give your body the energy that you need to burn out the muscle and the fuel that you need to replenish the muscle after you have burned it out. If you are not eating right and you are not refueling your body before and after your workouts, you are defeating the purpose of all your time at the gym. Basically, when you burn out your muscles, whether you are doing legs, arms, chest, back, abs, no matter what body part you are working on, you are depleting your muscles of the energy glycogen stores, or the glucose, otherwise known as the sugar in the muscles, when you feel the burn. You are tearing them down so they can rebuild themselves back up, therefore, making you stronger, leaner, and more defined. After you break the muscle fibers down or burn them out, it is imperative that you replenish what you have just depleted. You have to refuel and feed your muscles within thirty to forty-five minutes after your workout. You do this by consuming protein and simple carbohydrates. If you don't replenish the glycogen stores and protein your body could actually 'eat' your muscles for fuel, and you could potentially lose lean muscle mass? So make sure that you are consuming protein and carbs, especially post-workout. Remember protein is the building block of muscle, and now is the best time to start rebuilding muscle. Also remember that carbs are more important than you'll give them credit for, I'll guarantee it. Just make sure that you are eating the right carbs at the right time.

# TAKE A PILL, MAN!

Have you ever heard of a pill diet? No, not a diet pill. We all have heard of that! The fitness industry today is swamped with those. I am talking about a pill diet. One that would refer to the vitamins and supplements that one may take. Probably not unless you are a gym rat and you are continuously surrounded by lots of bodybuilders and fitness buffs. The fact of the matter is that you do not have to be any type of competitor or bodybuilder in order to utilize some kind of supplementation into your diet. Now when I speak of supplements, I am referring, at this moment in time, about the everyday person that may or may not have that strict of a diet. Let's face it people, we are all human, and we are all going to cheat on our new nutritional way of life. It is only necessary that we supplement with daily vitamins to ensure that we are giving our bodies all the nutrients that they need, to help us reach our ultimate goals, and to stay healthy and maintain that mode for the rest of our lives.

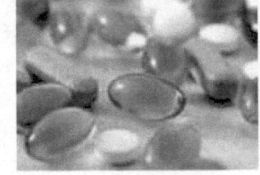

In the paragraphs to follow, I will explain to you some of what I perceive to be very beneficial supplements. You do not have to be a bodybuilder or fitness competitor to benefit from any of these. As I always say, though, please check with your health care professional or family physician before you add any of these supplements into your diet as they may have altering affects if you are taking any other medications.

First and foremost, I want to touch base on just your daily multivitamin. Believe it or not, there are so many people that are so into their physical training and do not take a multivitamin. Please take the time to find one that will work the best for you. I would recommend a multi that has a significant amount of nutrients and vitamins in it. One that may have everything from all the B-vitamins to Omega 3's and Vitamins A,C,D,E. Calcium, Potassium, and more. It is merely impossible to get all the nutrients that your body needs every day by what you consume. By taking in a multivitamin, you will add in the nutrients that you may be missing in your everyday diet.

A lot of people have asked me about EFAs. EFAs or (Essential Fatty Acids) are the building blocks of fats. Most EFAs are essential because we need them to live, yet our bodies cannot manufacture them on our own. We must ingest them by way of the foods that we eat. The word *essential* means "must be ingested." "Okay," you say, "so what do the Essential Fatty Acids actually do for me?" Well, believe it or not, this may take you by surprise; but they will benefit you in several different areas, such as:

- treating Eczema and maintaining healthy skin
- maintaining a healthy heart and arteries
- keeping cell membranes working properly and efficiently
- treating diabetic neuropathy
- relieving PMS and cyclical breast pain

You may not realize this, but you need EFAs to live. They are needed for maintaining proper cell membrane structure, which allows the nutrients from your diet to be properly distributed throughout your body and for efficient metabolism of cholesterol. EFAs are as essential as vitamins. If you do not get enough of them, you will become ill in some way. It has been shown that body cells that have been deprived of Essential Fatty Acids become cancerous, and it is difficult, if not impossible, to heal from cancer without adequate levels of these essential fats.

You can ingest EFAs from several different types of foods, including nuts, grains, and legumes; but you can also ingest them in an oil, pill, or capsule form. Flax seed above all is the highest, best quality of Omega-3 that can be ingested. It has been proven to lower cholesterol and also prevent the growth of new cancer cells.

One of my favorite supplements to take is, I gotta say, the B-Vitamins. B-Vitamins are truly a supplement that pinpoints so many different areas of your body. When you are deficient of B-Vitamins, so many things may be affected. Just take a look.

- **B1 (thiamine)**: Symptoms of this deficiency may include weakness in the limbs, insomnia, irregular heartbeat, edema (swelling of bodily tissues)
- **B2 (riboflavin)**: Deficiency may cause dry, cracked lips, high sensitivity to sunlight.
- **B3 (niacin)**: Deficiency may cause aggression, dermatitis, insomnia, weakness, mental confusion, and diarrhea.
- **B5 (pantothenic acid)**: Deficiency can result in acne.

- **B6 (pyridoxine)**: Deficiency may lead to anemia, depression, dermatitis, high blood pressure, Water retention, and hair loss. B-6 is also known as Biotin, as well as B-5 and B-7.
- **B7 (Biotin)**: Deficiency does not typically cause symptoms in adults but may lead to impaired growth and neurological disorders in infants.
- **B9 (folic acid)**: Deficiency in pregnant women can lead to birth defects. Research has also shown that folic acid might also slow the insidious effects of age on the brain.
- **B12 (cobalamin)**: Deficiency may cause memory loss and other cognitive deficits.

These are only a few examples of what some of the B-Vitamin family will do if you may be deficient in them. There are many wonderful advantages of taking the B-Vitamins:

- They support and increase the rate of metabolism
- Maintain healthy skin and muscle tone
- Enhance immune and nervous system function
- Promotes cell growth and division, including that of the red blood cells that help prevent anemia
- Reduce the risk of pancreatic cancer, one of the most lethal forms of cancer, when consumed with food, but not when ingested in vitamin tablet form
- And my favorite, they will give you that extra boost of energy, when it's needed in the middle of the day

All B-Vitamins are water soluble and are dispersed throughout the body. Most B-Vitamins must be replenished daily since any excess is excreted in the urine. Different B-Vitamins come from different food sources, such as liquid egg whites, potatoes, bananas, lentils, chili peppers, liver oil, liver, turkey, tuna, and Brewer's Yeast.

B-Vitamins may be injected or consumed in the pill form.

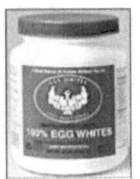 I had mentioned in a previous chapter the profound benefits of the Liquid Egg Whites. But remember, protein is the building block for muscle growth as well as helping in the battle against body fat. Liquid Egg Whites are the perfect source of protein for gastric bypass patients, athletes, world-class bodybuilders, and everyone in between. It is the best source of protein that anyone can consume or add into their daily diet. It is important to consume them throughout the day, but believe it or not,

the best time to take the Liquid Egg Whites is before bedtime. Fitness experts have known for decades that if you don't put protein into your body before you go to bed, your body will run out of protein in the middle of the night, causing your body to think that it is starving itself. To protect you, your body shuts down and starts storing your own fat cells. Your blood sugar still needs protein to keep you going, so it starts consuming the only protein source available at three o'clock in the morning, your own muscle mass. Basically, you are storing fat and eating muscle. By drinking a high protein drink with the Liquid Egg Whites just before you go to bed, the egg protein will support muscle growth for up to four to five hours. Now the process is reversed for most of your sleep time. Rather than storing fat and eating muscle, the protein from the egg whites is allowing your body to burn the fat at its normal rate while building on the muscle. You will get a better night's sleep, waking up more alert and refreshed, and yes, not as hungry in the morning. Now, after hearing that, who wouldn't want to add those into your diet? You would be crazy not to. Remember, though, it will only benefit you and your new nutritional way of life.

As we continue to move on into the book, we will get a little more in depth in a later chapter about what other supplements you may want to consider adding into your regimen should you decide to start training for a bodybuilding or fitness or figure competition. I would definitely recommend that you read everything, even if you are not planning to compete, only because, you may find that some of the supplements that will be mentioned in that particular chapter may spark a bit more interest in you and your journey.

# OH MY BACK!

Now, we're ready. I can remember when I first started weight lifting and doing resistance training. I topped out at 288 pounds, so when I first started my weight loss journey, I actually lived on ALL the cardio machines and watched my diet for a good twenty to twenty-five pounds, which took me about three months or so. It is actually very smart to start a great change with little changes at a time. I look at so many people that come into the gym, and I know in my heart of hearts, they have a long road ahead of them. What a lot of people don't realize is the fact that muscle weighs more than fat. Let me put it into perspective for you. Today, people have become so obsessed with the scale. If we work out for a week and we get on that scale and see that we have either lost nothing or stayed the same, we get so discouraged and say, "That's it! I quit. This is just a waste of time!" Listen, we are of the here and now. We see what we want, and we want it now. However, what so many people don't realize is that they are changing, but they are doing it from the inside out.

A young lady approached me one time in the gym, only to ask for advice. I saw myself in her shoes, how many years ago. Thinking that I was doing everything that I could do to try to transform my body, it just wasn't happening fast enough. She seemed a bit discouraged, overwhelmed so to speak, of all the weight equipment, cardio machines, the racks upon racks of weights, and dumbbells and proceeded to ask me, what would I advise her to do? I looked at her, only in amazement, knowing she is getting ready to go down the road less traveled. I knew what she was thinking and what she was feeling, and I responded, "Just stick with doing the cardio and cleaning up your diet for right now." I was not being mean. I was being dead serious. I knew where she was at. I have been there. It was very overwhelming, being in a position that she was really wanting to make a great change. So many people are not taught that muscle weighs more than fat, and I knew that if I had recommended to her that she started with certain weight equipment, she would definitely get discouraged because she would be changing from the inside out. The scale wasn't going to show her a significant weight loss at first, causing her to get discouraged and potentially quit. See, I was looking out for her best interest, and that was to encourage her to change her habits. Baby steps, my weary followers, baby steps.

I remember asking a trainer at the gym the same question. "What can I do to speed this up?" I was getting so discouraged. Her response, "Cardio and push-aways." "HUH?" I asked, I thought to myself, *What the heck are pushaway's? Cuz I am doing every kind of cardio, weight-lift, pull-up, pushback, tryin' to do push-ups, half squats, lunges, arm curls, you name it!* If I saw someone doing it, I was doing it too! But push-aways? "What are push-aways? I never heard of that?" She replied, "Push away from the table." I looked at her in utter amazement, like someone had smacked me in the head with a rubber tube. Duh, I knew that! Yeah, right! What I didn't realize at that time was that I was spending all my time doing all these exercises and cardio, and I **was** changing, slowly, but no one ever told me that muscle weighed more than fat; and no one ever told me that my diet was 80 percent of my transformation. So I wasn't seeing the change on the scale like I wanted to. Please remember this one very important thing. If you have never done any type of resistance training or weight lifting, when you start, and as you continue, YOU WILL PUT ON LEAN MUSCLE MASS, which means that you will not notice a significant amount of pounds lost on the scale, at first. But trust me when I say this, it will catch up to you, and you will begin to see those changes, so again, stay off the scale! Get yourself going in a new direction from your old habits and start slow. Change that nutritional way of life and get the cardio going good. Form those new habits of eating right and working out faithfully every day. Once you have those habits formed, then start adding in the resistance training and weight lifting.

What you will find in the pages to follow is only for when you are ready. A basic guideline to show you resistance training for every muscle group, a starting point, where you should be at the beginning of the exercise, and where you should be after a half rep. Your beginning and your end will be the same. As far as what days should you lift what body parts? That, my friend, is up to you; however, I have given you a sample week, just so you have a basic guideline. You only want to make sure that you don't lift the same body parts two days in a row, like biceps one day and triceps the next. Being that you wouldn't have arms two days in a row. Remember too, whenever you are doing a back exercise, most of the time you will also be using your biceps. Likewise, when you are doing chest, most of the time you will be using your triceps. You should train your abdominal muscles, just like every other muscle group. Every other day, you want to allow a day of rest in between to allow your muscles to fully repair themselves after you burn them out. Here's an example of a resistance training weekly workout. I would recommend this workout, if you are just starting to introduce resistance training into your daily regimen. If you are a bit more advanced, then you would want to really focus on one major muscle group every day.

MONDAY:        back, biceps, abs, and cardio
TUESDAY:       cardio
WEDNESDAY:     chest, triceps, abs, and cardio
THURSDAY:      cardio
FRIDAY:        shoulders, legs, abs, and cardio
Cardio should be at least 4 to 5 days a week 30 to 45 minutes.

For a more advanced workout schedule:

MONDAY:        chest and abs
TUESDAY:       back
WEDNESDAY:     legs and abs
THURSDAY:      shoulders
FRIDAY:        arms, biceps and triceps, and abs
Cardio should be at least 5 to 6 days a week 30 to 45 minutes.

*Back*

Low Rows:
    Hook band through the door anchor and place at the bottom of the door, close the door tight. Sit on the floor facing the door, with legs out in front of you. Move your arms forward and pull bands back squeezing your shoulder blades together, keeping your elbows close to your sides as you're pulling back. Make sure you are squeezing your shoulder blades together, like your holding a coin between your shoulder blades. Rowing motion, like you're a rowing a boat.

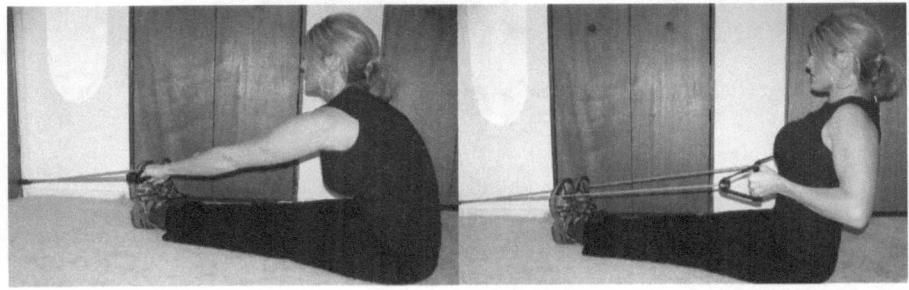

Lawn Mower pullbacks:

Standing on the middle of the band, take one handle in hand and pull arm back, like your starting a lawn mower. Make sure that you are squeezing your shoulder blade back. Switch arms and repeat with the other side.

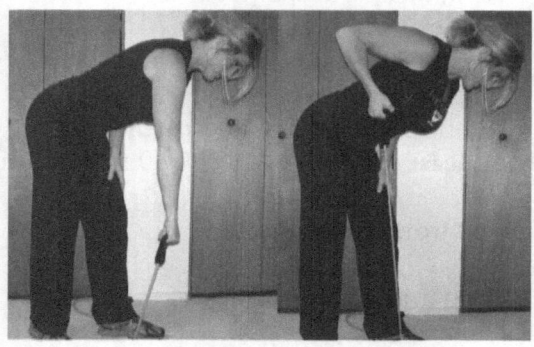

*Biceps*

Dumbbell curls:

Standing on the middle of the band, take both handles in hands and curl up, one arm at a time, keeping elbows by your side, really concentrating on flexing the bicep muscle.

Do not let the band pull your arms down; utilize the resistance with the band.

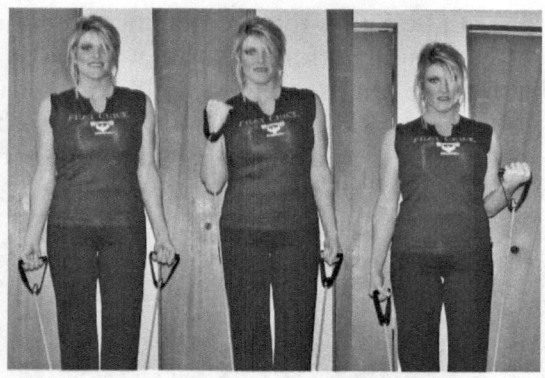

Straight bar curls:

Placing feet inside the handles of the band, hold band with both hands, keeping elbows by your side. Hold the band like a straight bar, curl up, again concentrating on flexing your biceps. Do not let the band pull your arms down; utilize the resistance with the band.

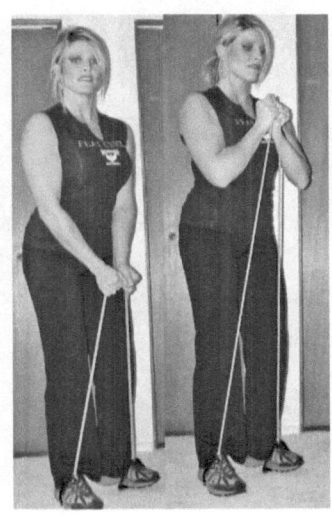

## Chest

High Flies:

Place the door anchor with the band at the top of the door. With your back to the door and standing about three to four feet from away, grab the band handles. With your arms out by your sides, elbows slightly bent and your body slightly bent over, pull the bands around to the front of you, like you're doing a big bear hug, squeezing and flexing your chest muscles.

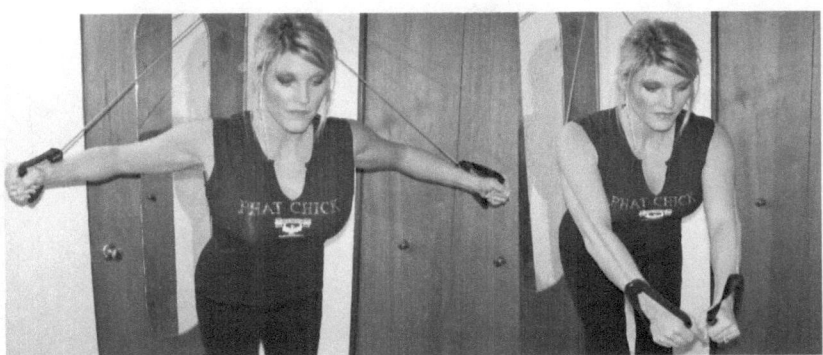

Countertop push-ups:

   In the push-up position, place your hands on the counter or a dresser, feet out about three to four feet away and do push-up, making sure that you again are squeezing your chest muscles as you come up.

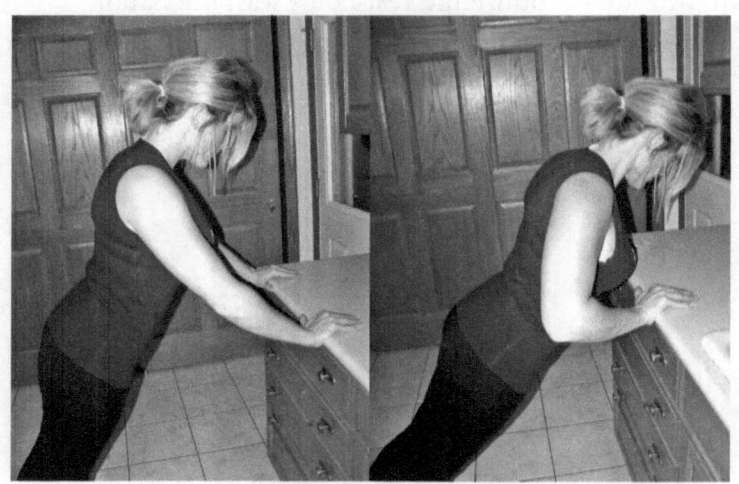

Low Flies:

   Place the door anchor with the band at the bottom of the door. With your back to the door and standing three to four feet away, grab the band handles. With your arms down and out by your sides and your body slightly bent over, pull the bands up to chest height, out in front of you, squeezing your chest muscles.

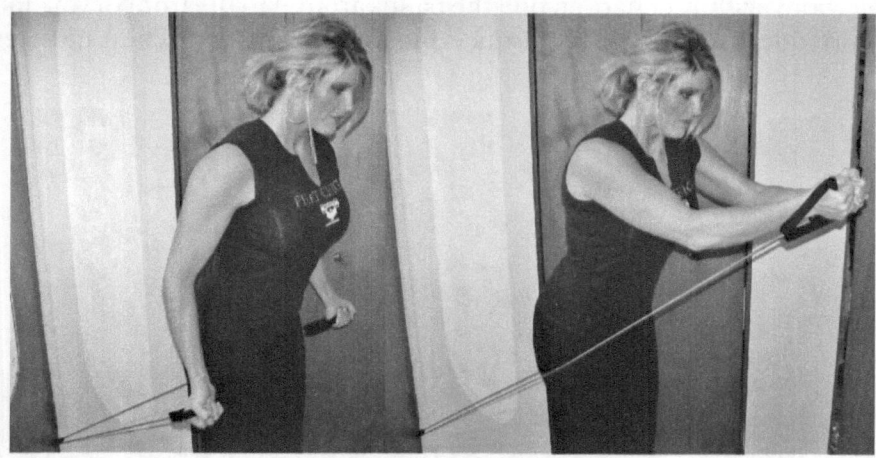

Chest Press:

With band inserted through door anchor and the anchor placed at the middle of the door, stand three to four feet away from the door, with your back to the door, pressing the bands straight out in front of you, flexing your chest as you press out.

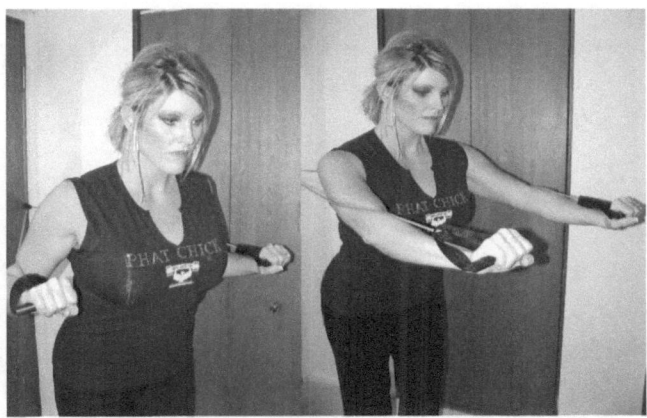

## Triceps

Overhead Triceps Extension:

Standing on the band, place your hand in the handle and pull the band up from behind your back. Keep your elbow close to your head, push arm up, moving only your elbow, focusing on flexing your triceps muscle.

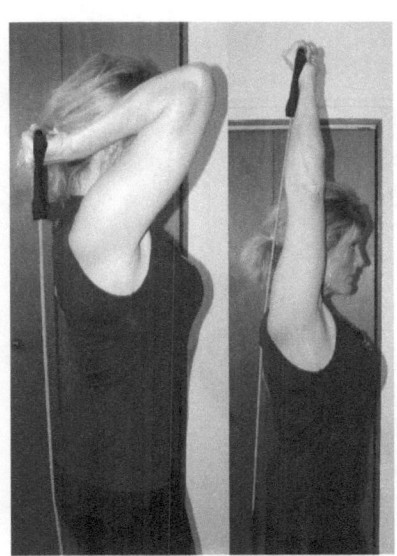

Triceps push-back:

With the band inside the door anchor and the anchor placed in the door at waist height, body bent over at a 90-degree angle with your elbow by your side. Bend your elbow only, pushing the band back. Don't use your shoulder or your arm to move the band. You should only be moving your elbow.

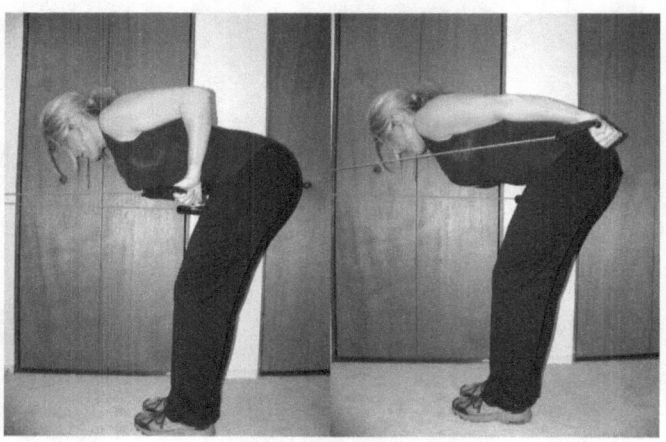

Triceps push-downs:

Place the door anchor at the top of the door, with the band through the anchor. Holding both handles of the bands, stand about three to five feet away from and face the door. Push the band down, utilizing the triceps muscles.

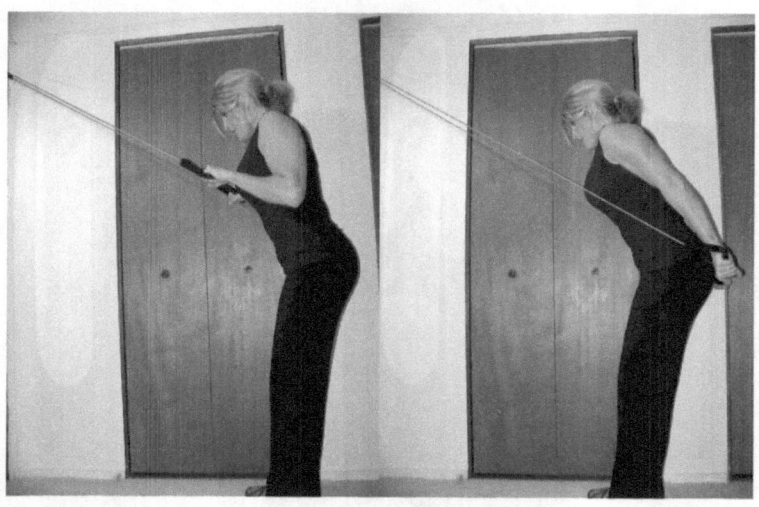

## Shoulders

Lateral Raises:
    Standing on the band, grab a hold of the handle. With elbow slightly bent, pull band straight out to your side, pulling it up. Remember to keep your elbow bent a little bit and use your shoulder muscle to pull the band up. Alternate your arms.

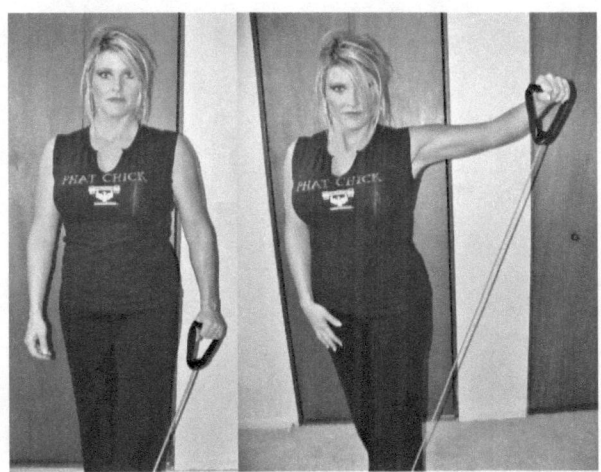

Upright rows:
    Standing with your feet in the handles of the band, grab the middle of the band, pull it up to your chin, and keep your elbows parallel with the floor as you're pulling up.

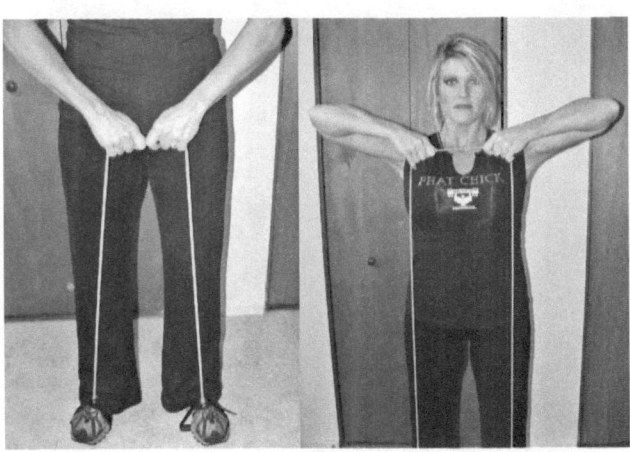

Shoulder presses:

Standing in the middle of the band, hands in handles, push the band up over your head.

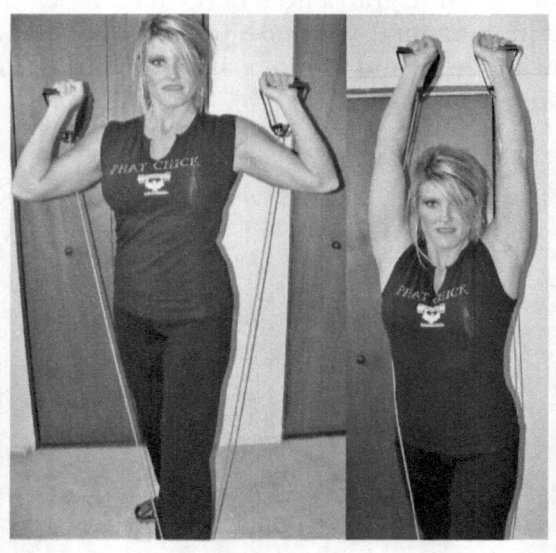

*Legs*

Counter Squats:

Stand next to the counter, holding onto the counter for balance only, squat down.

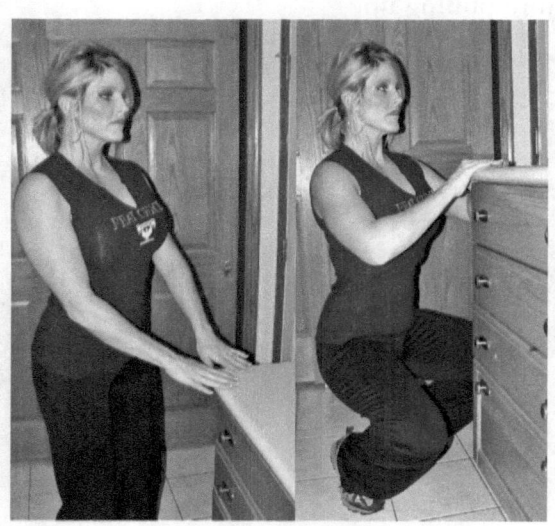

Squats:

    Standing in one place, squat down so knees are bent, back is straight, and legs are parallel to the floor, when you are down.

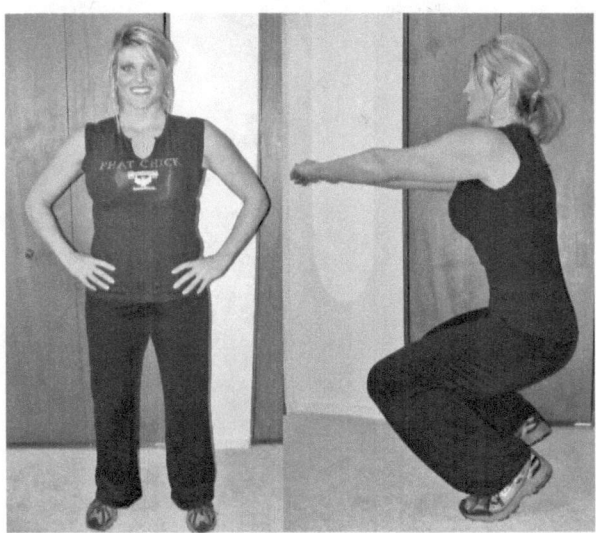

\*    For added resistance, stand with your feet in the middle of the band and, hands in handles, hold the bands parallel to your shoulders, and squat down.

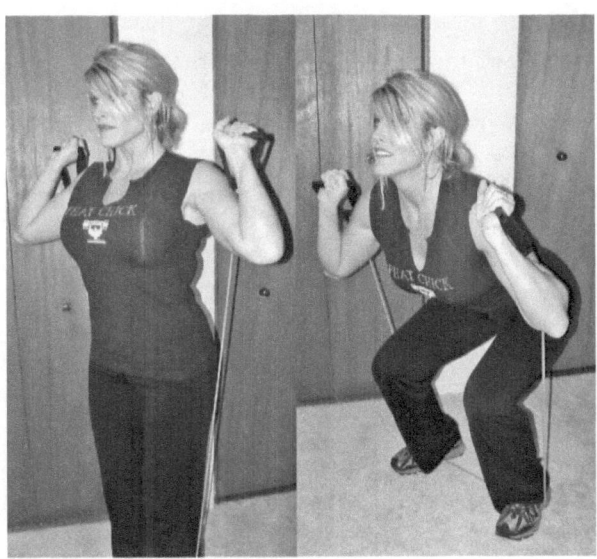

Standing Lunges:

Standing in one spot, lunge one leg at a time out in front of you, lunging back and forth.

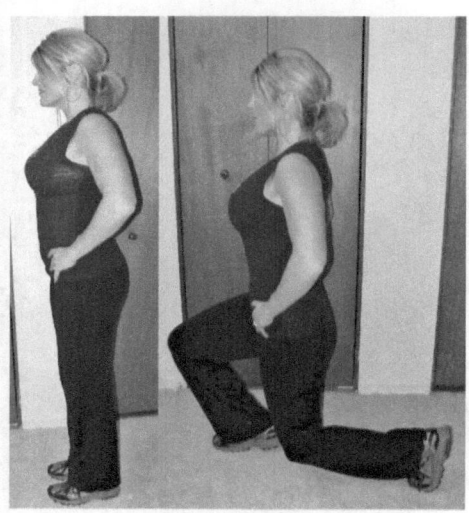

Hamstrings:

With the door anchor placed at the bottom of the door and the band pulled through, loop the band through each handle, forming a loop to place your foot through. With feet looped through each handle and your body facing the door, pull one foot up at a time, bending the knee. Work one leg at a time.

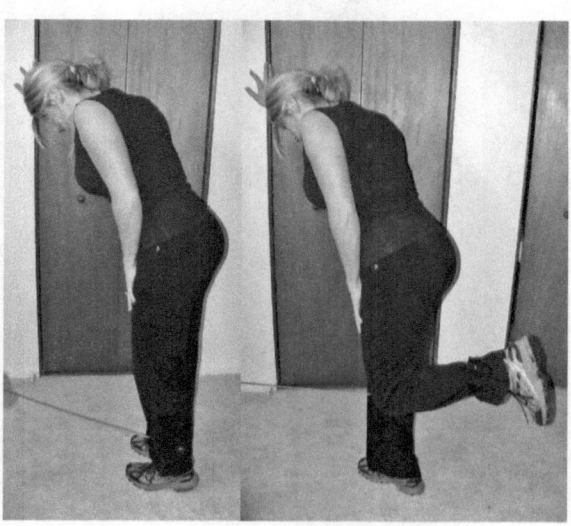

Glutes:

With the door anchor placed at the bottom of the door and the band pulled through, pull one handle through the other, securing the band at the anchor. Pull the band through the other handle, forming a loop to put your foot through. As with the hamstring exercises, keep body facing the door. This time, though, do not bend your knee up. Keep your knee slightly bent throughout the whole exercise and kick your leg straight back, really focusing on flexing your glute muscles.

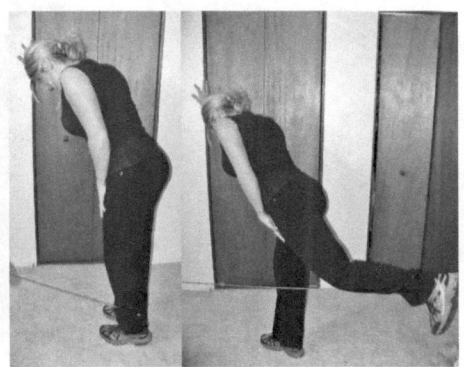

Kick Outs:

With the door anchor looped through and placed at the bottom of the door, pull one handle through the other, securing the band at the anchor. Pull the band through the other handle, forming a loop to put your foot through. Repeat the following exercises with each leg:

Outer Thighs:

Stand with your side to the door and kick your leg out, making sure to keep the band taut. Switch legs.

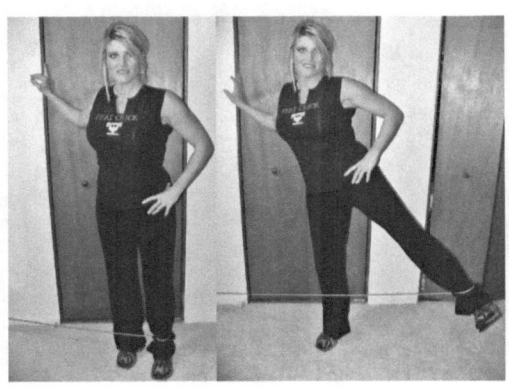

Inner Thighs:

Stand with your side to the door and pull your leg, kicking inward motion, making sure to keep the band taut. Switch legs.

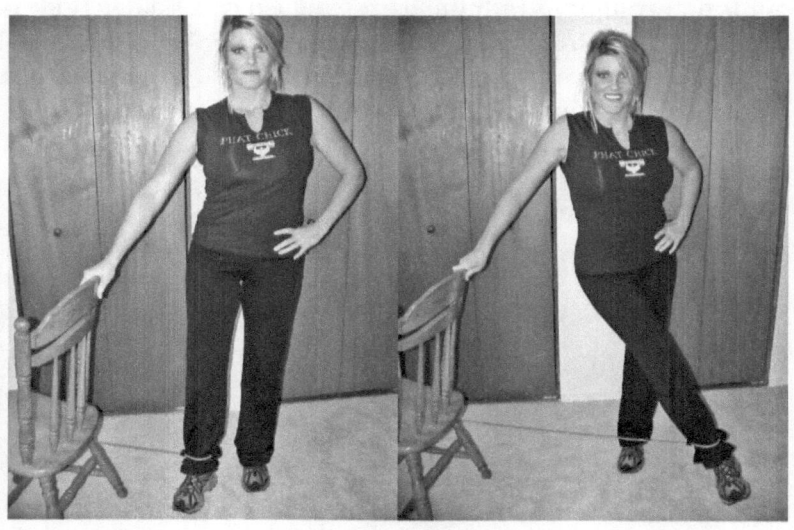

Quads:

Stand with your back to the door and pull your knee up, making sure to keep the band taut. Switch legs.

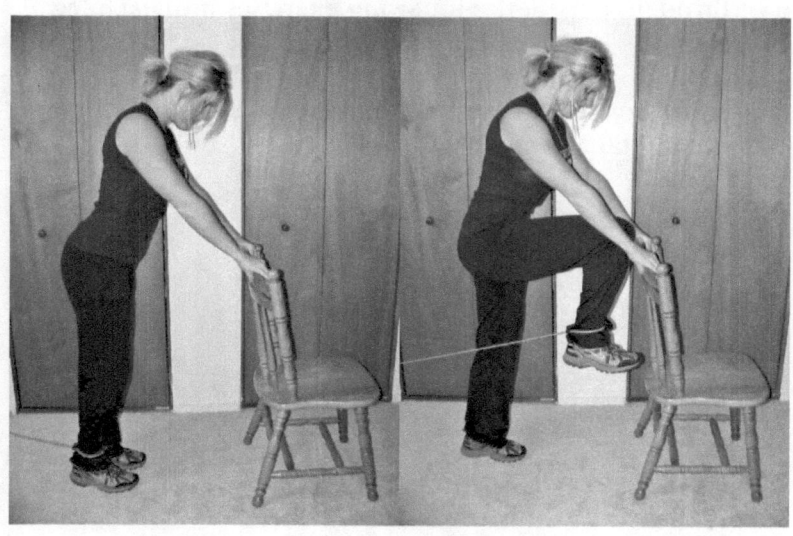

## *Ab Exercises*

These should be done with all three-workout days.

Crunches:
   Lying on the floor, knees bent, focus on a spot on the ceiling. Place your hands either behind your head, up to the ceiling, or over your chest, crunching up. Do not pull up on your neck. You want to pull your body up by using your abdominal muscles.

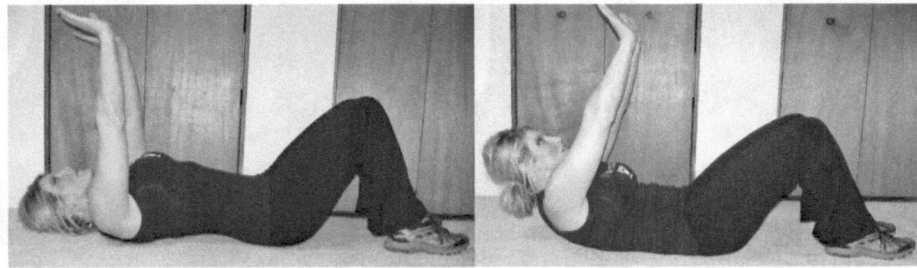

Crunches with added resistance:
   Just like the previous abs exercise, only now you add in the door anchor placed at the bottom of the door. Loop the band through the door. With your head closest to the door and your body about two to four feet away, grab the handles of the band and hold your arms straight down by your sides. Pull your body up now, by just using your abdominal muscles again.

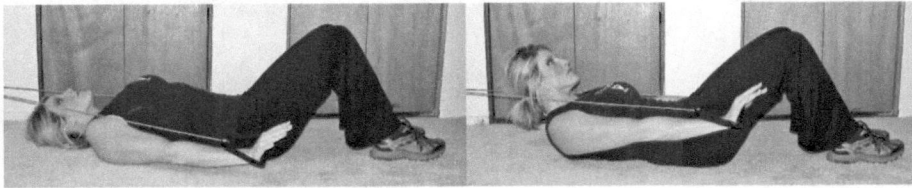

Leg Lifts:

Lying flat on the floor, with your legs out in front of you and knees slightly bent, bring your legs straight up from your body and then down again. Do not let your feet touch the floor. For an extra challenge, hold them two to three inches above the floor and hold the position for ten to twenty second intervals.

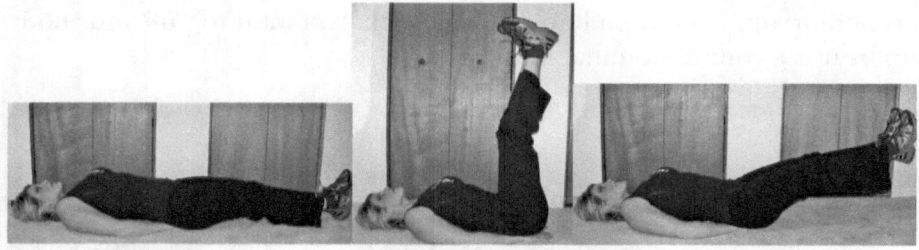

Obliques:

In the crunches position, lie with your back flat on the floor. Twist your legs to one side, with your knees together. Hold this position and crunch up, remembering to not pull on your neck. Squeeze up with your oblique muscles and then repeat on each side.

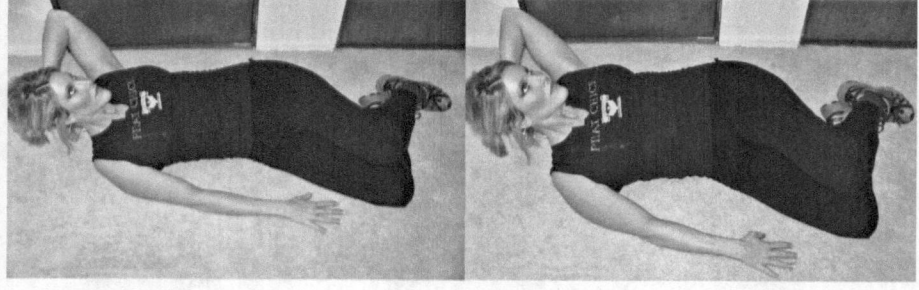

# MUSCLE HEADS

When it comes to competing, it takes so much dedication. There aren't enough words in the dictionary to explain the heart of a person that decides to compete and follows through with it. The time, and the preparation that goes into training, and the diet alone are unbelievable. I never realized the mental strength that it takes to actually do it. Several years ago, I had this thought in my head that I would love to compete one day. I wanted to picture myself as that muscular, fitness chick up on that stage, in all my glory, just posing away and flaunting my stuff! Although when I looked in the mirror, the only thing that I would have qualified for at that time would have been a hot dog-eating contest. And the Lord knows I would have won, and still to this day, I could eat the best of them under the table! This old girl can chow down. But, in all honesty, when I finally reached the point in my weight loss and transformation journey, I didn't realize the passion that one has to have for that sort of training and dedication. I have definitely learned, and give great respect for those who do compete.

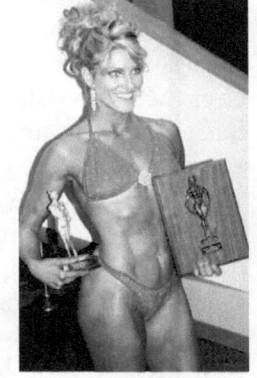

Almost five years to the day when I walked into my first weight-loss meeting, I stepped on stage for the first time. I cannot explain the emotional

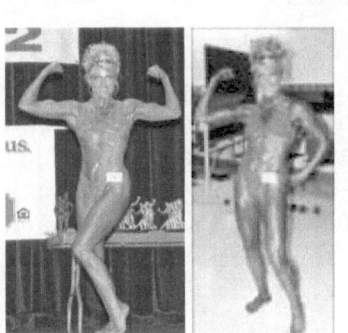

buildup that went through my mind right up to the second before I was to step on stage. Being as heavy as I once was, I often still pictured myself overweight. That being said, you can imagine the nervousness that I experienced when I put on that little bitty suit and six-inch high heels and looked out into the audience, trying to put myself in a place that I never thought that I would be. Not only overcoming the fear of being in

47

front of an audience and judges, but putting myself in a place where I would actually allow innocent bystanders to look at me in that skimpy little suit and judge me. I must have been crazy! And you know what, I still am! It took one time, and I am so hooked. I had the best time up on that stage. Words cannot ever express the feeling of accomplishment that I had at that moment. I had done it, and I had worked my butt off doing it, but you know what? It was all worth it in the end. What I am trying to say is that if you have ever thought of competing but never really thought you could do it, DO IT! When that thought first enters your mind and you truly believe that you can do it, YOU CAN! I tell everyone, if I can do it, anybody can. But just be prepared to give it 150 percent. I promise in the end you will have the most gratifying feeling of accomplishment. Whether you win or not, if you finished the race to the stage, you really did win.

So where do you start? Well, in order to compete, my first advice would be that you really need to be in remotely good shape. Have your body fat, weight, measurements, and lean body mass done, by either a family doctor or a personal trainer. You should find a nutritionist that can personalize a diet for you and help you prepare and change your diet every so often. I would definitely suggest, for your first show, that you plan on starting your training and cleaning up your diet about sixteen weeks out. Don't leave room for time to cut you short. Give it your all, and give it all you got. When you are dieting for competition, it

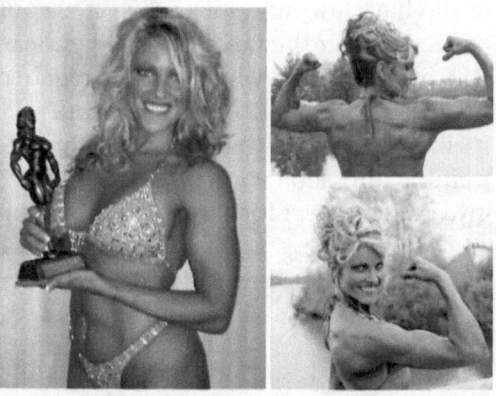

is imperative that you do NOT cheat at all on your diet. It truly has to be immaculate. Think about it like this, though, it is only four months. In reality, that is not that long, especially for such an accomplishment.

Make sure that you start adding in special supplements to your diet. You will be depriving your body of some nutrients, and you will also be cutting more body fat and adding more lean muscle. There are several supplements that I always add into my pill diet when I am training for competition. I also add in extra protein and supplemental powders to my shakes, including 100 percent Pure Liquid Egg Whites in place of water. The following is a list of all the benefits of adding these into your regimen and why. Again, you should always consult your family physician before adding any new supplements into your diet as they may have altering effects should you be taking any other medication.

- **Protein Shakes:** I use Whey Isolate protein mixed with liquid egg whites in my daily shakes. Occasionally I will also use soy isolate protein-based products as the soy base is not as harsh on the belly as whey sometimes may be. The main thing is to use the liquid egg whites in place of water or milk. Because the liquid egg whites are 100 percent bio-available for four to five hours, and the powders are only about 70 percent bio-available for two to three hours. I save money on my powders by using half as much and getting twice as many shakes per bottle. More bang for my buck. Powders are getting very expensive. But by cutting the powders in half and mixing with the liquid egg whites, I get 20 percent more protein in my body for two hours longer than I would by just using the powders alone. I use the protein shakes as my meal 3 and 5, along with a simple carb on meal 3 (that's normally after my workout). Before bedtime, I drink mostly the liquid egg whites protein. I have done a lot of research in comparison of the whey and the soy protein, curious on which is prospectively better. My findings are as follows: Soy protein is actually just as good as the whey. I perceive that the soy protein shakes would be better to consume post-workout. As they, just like the whey, provide "**some**" essential amino acids to help your muscles recover; however, the soy-based protein will also help with muscle soreness and inflammation. The liquid egg whites are an all-natural food and a complete protein that supplies "**all**" of the essential amino acids, unlike protein supplement powders, which are incomplete proteins. My advice is if you are going to utilize a soy-based protein, do a fifty-fifty whey/soy protein shake post-workout, mixing with 100 percent pure liquid egg whites. Adding your protein with the liquid egg whites will enhance your protein intake up to an extra 20 percent of protein from the egg whites, depending on how many ounces you are using. I recommend eight ounces per drink. When putting on muscle mass, it is important to know your lean body mass. We talked a bit about this in a previous chapter, but remember, your basic calculation for gaining muscle is 1.5g of protein x (your total lean body mass). So if your LBM (lean body mass) is 150 pounds, you multiply that by 1.5, which is 225. This means that you should take in 225g of protein a day to increase your muscle mass.
- **Glutamine:** Decreases your muscle recovery time, increases endurance after a depletion in glycogen stores from that burning out, decreases your chances of illness by boosting your immune system, and helps prevent overtraining from long workout activity.
- **Glucosamine with Chondritin:** Supports and lubricates your joints, which is definitely needed when you are doing a lot of strenuous lifting

and training. Glucosamine with Chondritin can be formulated with another ingredient called MSM (or Methylsulfonylmethane)—yeah, try pronouncing that one! It actually helps with joint pain. You see, MSM is a sulfonyl sulfur that is found in the fluid and tissues of all living organisms. It's also a component of structural protein, the type found in hair, skin, and joints. Sulfur also occurs in connective tissue or cartilage, therefore, aiding in joint pain.

- **Calcium:** Helps support and keep your bones strong, but it also helps you relax your muscles and with the cramping.
- **Vitamin C:** Helps keep your immune system strong. When you are training all the time, it is imperative that you continue to take all of your daily vitamins as your immune system may suffer from overtraining.
- **CLA (Conjugated Linoleic Acid):** Helps increase muscle mass while reducing body fat. It is also an antioxidant and helps the immune system, which is extremely important with a high-intensity training program.
- **L-Carnitine:** Helps metabolize food into energy, also helps with fat burning, increasing energy, and improving resistance to muscle fatigue. Also reduces feelings of hunger and weakness.

I am sure that there are a million and one supplements that you could also add into your training program, but my best advice is that you honestly research whatever you want to take and make sure that you talk to your nutritionist and your family physician. Choose a competition date and run for the fences! The sky is the limit, and you can sincerely do anything that you put your heart, soul, and mind into doing! Best of luck to you, but just go for it!

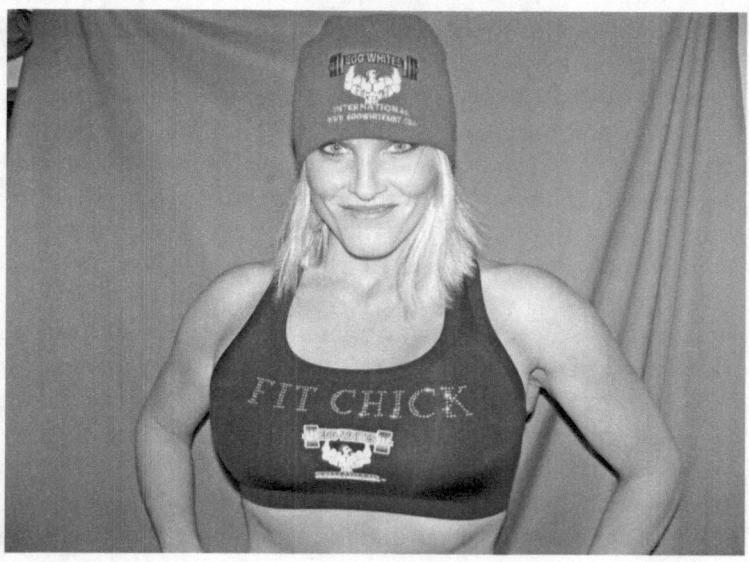

# WHICH CAME FIRST, THE CHICKEN OR THE EGG?

I have used several different supplements throughout my weight loss journey, and I have tried it all. But let me just say, as mentioned periodically throughout previous chapters, Liquid Egg Whites from Egg Whites International, has enriched my daily nutritional life. Unfortunately, I didn't discover Egg Whites International until I was already in the middle of my weight loss journey. Had I known then what I know now, I would have been utilizing them in my everyday diet. I highly recommend Egg Whites International to all of my clients, regardless of weight-loss or whatever their circumstances may be. The benefits that I have acquired with them not only in my diet, my children's diets, and with my clients' progress have been endless. There were so many times that it was time to eat, and I was scrambling around, searching for that "in between" meal. I found, that eight ounces of liquid egg whites was filling, yet it was also quick, and I was getting more protein in my daily life. I could literally grab it and go. The following chapter is an insert that a dear friend of mine wrote. I asked Mac if he could just write about the true benefits of what the egg whites can really do for everyone. I am so grateful for his input, but more thankful that I was given the opportunity to actually find a product that truly has changed my life.

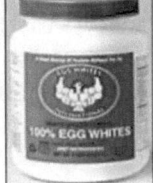 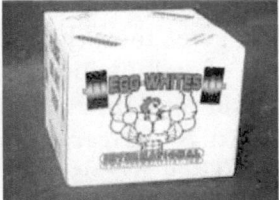

# EGG WHITES ARE NATURE'S PERFECT FOOD!

## What You Really Need to Know

Egg Whites have always been considered to be the perfect all-natural food protein. Egg White Albumen is used in flu shots and most commonly in IVs in hospitals when you are laid up and not eating solid foods. Doctors always refer to Egg Whites as Albumen. Ask one sometime and see what they say. When you go to get a flu shot, they always ask if you have any allergies to eggs because you can't get a flu shot if you do.

Egg Whites are also one of the only 100 percent Bio-available and complete proteins in the world. They have a complete essential amino acid profile, unlike protein powders, which are considered incomplete proteins. When protein powders are rated on the BV rating, they are always compared to how they stand up against egg white protein. On a scale of 1 to 10, with 10 being best, Egg Whites are always the 10 on every scale. Liquid egg whites are higher on the scale than powdered egg whites.

Doctors today are looking for better sources of protein to help people with severe health problems like cancer, diabetes, malnutrition—you name it. In fact, most cancer doctors will tell you that a lot of people with cancer die of malnutrition and not just cancer. Because the chemotherapy tends to kill your appetite and cause vomiting, it is very hard to keep solid foods down. So cancer patients tend to lose weight. But they are not just losing fat. They are also losing muscle. Doctors will suggest protein drinks to help patients get ample amounts of protein that they can keep in their stomach while fighting cancer. But, most all of, these protein drinks are inferior to 100 percent pure liquid egg white protein. They have a lot of fillers and sugars. Some are good and some are hype. Doctors are just now starting to find out about Egg Whites International to recommend to their patients. Gastric bypass, lap band, and bariatric doctors are also starting to recommend this to their patients as well.

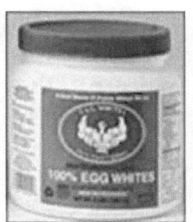

Egg Whites International's 100 percent Pure Liquid Egg Whites are the only liquid egg white on the market that is primarily sold as a drink. Every other egg white product on the market is sold for baking or cooking. Egg Whites International has taken the extra steps to basically reinvent the egg. By pasteurizing and double filtering the egg white to remove the slimy texture, they created the perfect protein drink. Liquid egg whites taste like water, with a slight saltwater taste because of the natural and minimal amount of sodium found in egg whites. However, they take on the flavor of whatever you mix them with. Want lemonade? Take a cup of liquid egg whites, add some powder lemonade mix, and you have pure protein lemonade. Use your imagination.

For decades, there has been a catch 22 about egg whites. They are the world's most perfect protein in the raw state, but your body can't digest a raw egg white because of Avidin, found in raw egg whites. Avidin blocks your vitamin B6 uptake, causing a Biotin deficiency. You must cook the egg white to neutralize the Avidin, making them useable for the human body to utilize the proteins. However, by cooking the egg whites to be able to digest them, you overcook them and denature the protein. You lose about 12 percent of the available protein, so you no longer have the world's perfect protein at 100 percent. Hence, catch 22. You can't get there from here.

Something more that we have heard from several of our clients, is that their hair has gotten thicker since they started using the liquid egg whites. Men, because their hair is typically shorter than women, for the most part, are getting haircuts more often, because their hair is growing faster and thicker than before. Now I am not suggesting that Liquid Egg Whites are a hair growth product by any means. So, please don't go buy a bunch of liquid egg whites if your bald or losing your hair and expect to get your hair back, that's not what I am trying to promote. The fact is that hair is pure protein. So basically any increase in protein, even fish or chicken in your diet should have the same effect. So it makes sense that an increase of protein in your diet would help support hair protein. The protein from egg whites is just easier to absorb and is also good for skin, nails, muscle growth and fat burning. For decades, before hair conditioners came on the market, they would crack and egg and use the egg whites for hair conditioner in salons. Some salons still do today. They would also take an egg white and some lemon juice and use it on your face, to let it dry for a facial. The old days are not so far behind us! We learn from our ancestors.

In the movie *Rocky*, he drinks a whole raw egg. This works somewhat because egg yolks are loaded with Biotin. So, by drinking both the raw egg white and the yolk, your body can digest about 30 percent of the available protein, but not much more because it is still a raw egg. The Biotin in the yolk offsets the Avidin in the egg white to give some balance. Raw eggs are still not healthy to drink raw because of the threat of *Salmonella* and *Listeria*. Not to mention they taste like raw eggs.

Children with ADD, night terrors, and just bad eating habits benefit from egg whites as well. Keep in mind that proper nutrition is the basic structure of how well we live our lives and the quality of life we live. Healthier is better. And what better way to start than with your kids' health.

This was a letter sent to us after recommending Egg Whites International to a client.

### *"MY CHILDREN ARE HEALTHIER!"*

> We started using Egg Whites International for my two-year-old son who has multiple eating (or lack of eating) problems and had great success with him. So we decided to also give your liquid egg whites to my four-year-old daughter who had night terrors on a fairly regular basis, which doctors could not explain. Immediately her night terrors stopped. My daughter now sleeps through the night and wakes up happy, and this has been consistent ever since we started supplementing her diet with Egg Whites International.

> In addition, my son who is allergic to the "crack your own eggs" has no problem with Egg Whites International at all. Both my children are healthier by adding this product to their drinks. As a mom, I have peace of mind knowing my children are using a safe and beneficial supplement. Thank you, Egg Whites International!

# FEED MY BELLY

I've included in this chapter an array of different recipes, ideas, and tips to help in your new nutritional way of life. You will find at the end of each recipe a serving size and nutrient guide for any type of diet. Remember, though, the sky is the limit when it comes to your eating habits. Any recipes that you may have at home can be altered to become a bit healthier. It is when you stop living to eat and start eating to live that you will become more aware of what you are putting in your body and in your families' bodies.

## *BREAKFAST RECIPES*

### *KELLI'S HOMEMADE PROTEIN PANCAKES*

5 egg whites
1/2 cup quick dry oatmeal
Sprinkle cinnamon
2-3 packets Splenda

In a blender, mix all ingredients, blend to a pancake consistency. While mixing up the ingredients, start warming your pan. Spray with a noncook spray and heat on medium heat. Drop mixture into pan, forming your own size pancakes. Cook 1-2 minutes on each side or until golden brown. Remove from heat. Top with either sugar-free syrup, reduced fat peanut butter, and sugar-free jelly. Or just butter spray with a sprinkle of more cinnamon and Splenda. Please note that adding the peanut butter, jelly, or sugar-free syrup will alter the nutrient contents in this recipe.

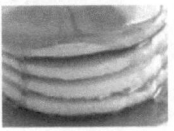

Serving Size: Entire Mixture
  190 calories
  19g protein
  22g carbs
  2g fat

*use 'pancake' as a protein wrap, just remove splenda and cinnamon from recipe.

## *PEANUT BUTTER MAPLE OATMEAL*

1/2 cup quick dry oatmeal
1 cup water
1 tablespoon reduced fat peanut butter
1 teaspoon brown sugar Splenda

In a microwave safe bowl, mix dry oats and water. Microwave on high until oatmeal is cooked to your desired consistency. Add in peanut butter and brown sugar Splenda. Mix up and enjoy!

    Serving Size:  1 cup
                      170 calories
                      6.5g protein
                      21g carbs
                      7.5g fat

## *PUMPKIN PIE OATMEAL*

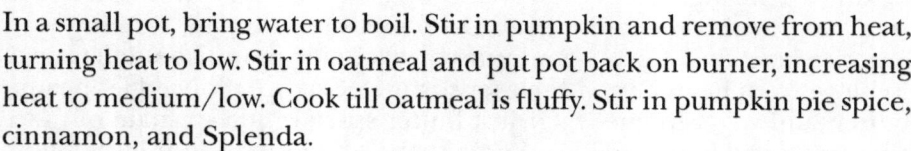

1 cup water
1/2 can pumpkin
1/2 cup quick dry oatmeal
1 tablespoon cinnamon
1 teaspoon pumpkin pie spice
2 tablespoons Splenda

In a small pot, bring water to boil. Stir in pumpkin and remove from heat, turning heat to low. Stir in oatmeal and put pot back on burner, increasing heat to medium/low. Cook till oatmeal is fluffy. Stir in pumpkin pie spice, cinnamon, and Splenda.

    Serving Size:  1 cup
                      110 calories
                      4g protein
                      23g carbs
                      6g fiber
                      2g fat

## MEXICAN MORNING PIZZA

1 low-fat, whole wheat wrap
1 whole egg
1 egg white
1/4 bell pepper, diced
1/4 onion, diced
1/2 cup salsa
1/4 cup shredded part-skim mozzarella cheese

Preheat oven to 350 degrees, place wrap on a baking sheet, and cook, flipping halfway through for 10 minutes. Meanwhile, in a small bowl, scramble egg and egg white. Spray your pan with nonstick cooking spray. Add pepper and onion and sauté for about 5 minutes until soft. Add in your egg mixture and cook, stirring often until set. Remove your wrap from the oven, place the salsa on top of the tortilla, then the egg mixture, and top off with the cheese. YUMMY!

Serving Size:  1 tortilla
               325 calories
               22g protein
               31 g carbs
               5g fiber
               12 g fat

Remember that when you are planning your nutritional plan, you want a variety. Try not to eat the same things every day. When you allow yourself to get stuck in the rut of eating the same things every day, you are not teaching yourself to live life, and your body will be more susceptible to plateauing quicker. There is NO way that you are going to be able to eat the same thing every day for the rest of your life! Variety is very important, and you are not going to want to deprive yourself of the things that you love. So let's just find alternatives, so we don't have to miss out on one of the best things in life—food!

As I continue, I am going to give you some more recipes for lunches and dinners and even some snacks. But remember, you can alter any recipe that you may find, by just changing up some of the ingredients to make them better for you in general. For example, ground beef can be substituted with ground sirloin, ground turkey, or ground chicken. Butter can be substituted with no-calorie, no-fat butter spray. Sugar can be substituted with sweetener, such as Splenda. Salt may be substituted with Mrs. Dash or any other leading brand of no-sodium or salt-free seasoning. Read your labels. When you are grocery shopping, just take that extra minute or two and see what you are exactly putting in your body. The more salt that you have in your diet, the more likely you are to retain water. It is little changes in your diet and everyday life that will have the better long-term effects in your overall health.

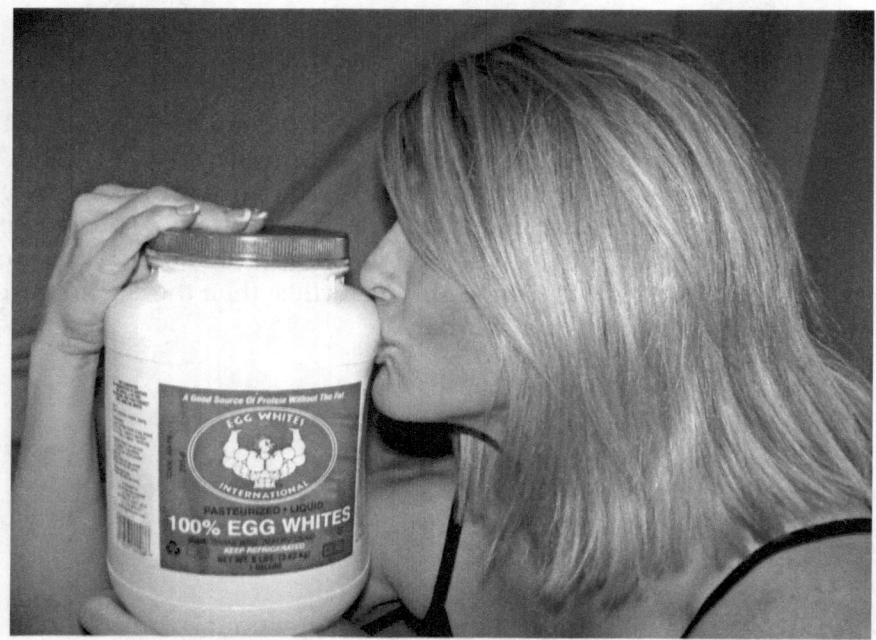

# LUNCHES AND DINNERS

## CHICKEN AND RICE

5 ounces of cooked boneless, skinless, chicken breast
1/4 cup brown rice
1/2 cup water
1 cup fresh broccoli salt-free seasoning

Shred the chicken breast and place aside. In a microwavable safe bowl, add in water, rice, and broccoli. Place a lid over the mixture and microwave on high until rice is fully cooked and broccoli has been steamed to soft texture, about 5-7 minutes, depending on your microwave. Remove and add the mixture and add in the shredded chicken breast and some of your favorite seasonings and butter spray. Place mixture back in the microwave for about 2 minutes to heat the chicken through. Remove and enjoy.

Serving Size: One bowl
204.5 calories
33g protein
16.5g carbs
1g fat

## *PROTEIN PASTA*

1 teaspoon olive oil
1 cup chopped onion
1 pound lean ground turkey breast
2 cups broccoli florets
1 cup chopped fresh plum tomatoes
2 teaspoons tomato paste
1 tablespoon low-sodium tamari
3/4 teaspoon minced garlic
2 cups nonfat cottage cheese, divided
2 cups brown rice shell pasta, cooked and divided
1 teaspoon each sea salt and ground white pepper, divided
1 tablespoon low-fat grated Parmesan cheese, (optional)

Preheat oven to 350 degrees. In a large skillet, heat olive oil over med-high heat. Add onion and turkey. Cook until turkey is no longer pink. Add broccoli, tomato, tomato paste, tamari, and garlic and stir while cooking for 5 more minutes or until broccoli is bright green. Remove from heat. Place a layer of turkey mixture in the bottom of a casserole dish and top with a layer of cottage cheese, a layer of pasta, and a dusting of both sea salt and pepper. Repeat the layers, like a lasagna dish, until all ingredients have been used up. Top with Parmesan cheese if desired. Bake uncovered for 30 minutes or until golden brown on top.

Serving Size:   Entire dish makes 4-5 servings.
                360 calories
                45g protein
                35g carbs
                1g fat
                8g fiber

## *TURKEY AND VEGGIE MEATLOAF*

3/4 cup water or low-sodium chicken broth
3/4 cup finely diced sweet onion
3/4 cup diced plum tomatoes
1 pound lean ground turkey breast
1/4 cup diced green pepper
1/4 cup diced red pepper
1 cup oat bran
1 teaspoon dried celery flakes
1/2 teaspoon ground sage
1/2 teaspoon dried thyme
2 teaspoon Worcestershire sauce
1/2 teaspoon black pepper
3 egg whites

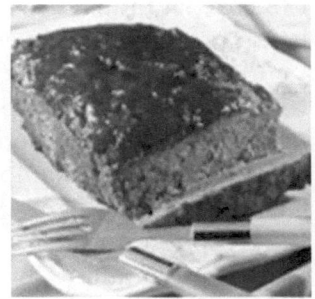

Preheat oven to 350 degrees. In a small skillet, heat water or broth and sauté onion and broccoli until onion is translucent. Add tomatoes and remove from heat. In a mixing bowl, combine remaining ingredients. Add vegetable mixture and mix thoroughly. Lightly spray a loaf pan with olive oil and pat mixture into pan. Bake for 40 minutes or until golden brown. Slice and serve with additional steamed broccoli and tomatoes.

Serving Size: Loaf makes 4-5 servings
210 calories
33g protein
20g carbs
3g fat
5g fiber

# DESSERTS AND TREATS

## SWEET POTATO MUFFINS WITH FLAX AND BRAN

1/3 cup oat bran
1/3 cup ground flax seed
1 cup whole wheat flour
1-1/2 teaspoon baking powder
1/2 teaspoon baking soda
1-1/2 teaspoon cinnamon
1-1/2 teaspoon ginger
1/2 teaspoon nutmeg
1/2 teaspoon salt
2/3 cup brown sugar Splenda
2 cups cooked mashed sweet potatoes
2 tablespoons olive oil
1-1/3 cups buttermilk
4 egg whites
1-1/2 teaspoon vanilla
3/4 cup pitted dates, chopped

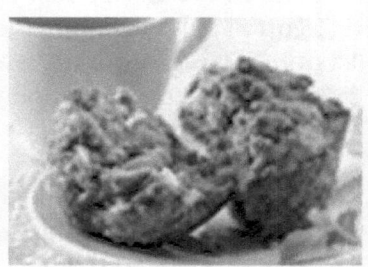

Preheat oven to 400 degrees. Spray 24 muffin cups with nonstick spray. In a large bowl, combine oat bran, flax, flour, baking powder, baking soda, cinnamon, ginger, nutmeg, salt, and sugar. In a separate bowl, whisk together sweet potatoes, oil, buttermilk, eggs, and vanilla. Stir sweet potato mixture into dry ingredients just until moistened. Stir in dates. Divide among 24 muffin cups. Bake for about 20 minutes or until done.

Serving Size:  1 muffin
                  105.8 calories
                  2.9g protein
                  20.1g carbs
                  2.5g fat
                  2.5g fiber

## *STRAWBERRY CHEESECAKE DESSERT*

4 ounces fat-free Ricotta
1/2 dry package Jell-O sugar-free Cheesecake Pudding
1 cup 1 percent milk
3/4 cup Cool Whip FREE
2 cups Fresh Strawberries, halved
4 teaspoons Splenda

Wash and halve fresh strawberries into a bowl. Add 4 teaspoons of Splenda and mix lightly. Set aside.

In a blender, add:

4 ounces fat-free Ricotta
1/2 dry package Jell-O SF Cheesecake Pudding
1 cup nonfat milk

Blend until thick and creamy. Pour into clean bowl and add Cool Whip FREE. Fold gently. Spoon a little pudding mixture into pudding dish, add a couple strawberries, and keep layering until you've used 1/4 of the pudding mix per serving. Top with remaining strawberries. Enjoy!

Serving Size:  4
              90.5 calories
              4.9g protein
              17.3g carbs
              0.4g fat

## *HOMEMADE PEANUT BUTTER FUDGE PROTEIN BARS*

4 scoops chocolate whey protein isolate powder
2/3 cup flax seed meal
4 tablespoons natural reduced fat peanut butter
1/4 cup water
Splenda (optional)
2 tablespoons cocoa powder (optional)

Mix all ingredients in a large bowl and stir. At first it may not seem like it has enough water, but keep stirring and it will eventually become a sticky blob of dough. Add 1 tablespoon of water at a time if needed.

Divide mixture into 4 equal portions and place in separate pieces of plastic wrap, placing them into bars. It's easier to shape them by lying plastic wrap on one side of a small casserole dish, pressing the dough into the natural shape of the dish. Store the bars in fridge or freezer. Once solid, enjoy.

    Serving Size:  1 bar
                         280.7 calories
                         28g protein
                         13.5 carbs
                         14.1g fat
                         8.9g fiber

**Some extras on the recipe end. Liquid Egg White Recipes . . . What can you really do with the Liquid Egg Whites from Egg Whites International? Take a look, the sky is the limit.**

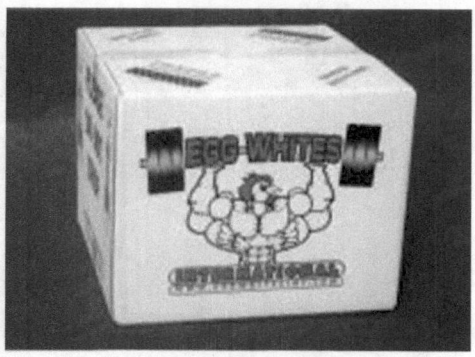

# QUICK PROTEIN DRINK IDEAS

Here are some quick and easy high protein drinks with items you may already have in your refrigerator at home. Ideas from our customers to share with you.

Take one eight-ounce cup of our 100 percent pure liquid egg whites (26g protein) and mix with any of the following liquids for a fast meal replacement. No blender, just a shaker cup or stir well.

Fat-free or sugar-free "liquid" coffee creamers make great drinks. Coffee Mate and International Delight have lots of great flavors. These are concentrated, so a 2-ounce serving is plenty with 8 ounces of Liquid Egg Whites. You can also add 2 ounces of milk for a 12-ounce drink.

Suggested coffee creamers to use with 8oz of Liquid Egg Whites include:

2 ounces **Southern butter pecan** (This would be great at bedtime.)
2 ounces **pumpkin pie spice** (Seasonal item, very good.)
2 ounces **french vanilla** or **hazelnut**
2 ounces **chocolate caramel** (This is hard to find, but this is very good.)

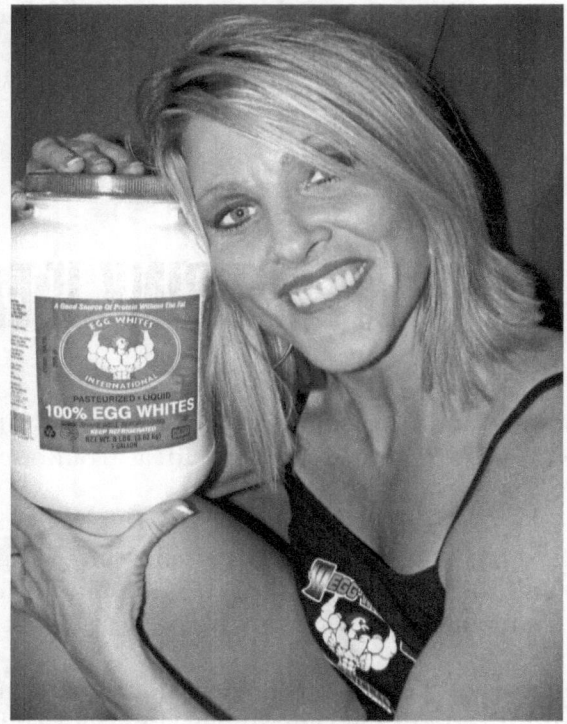

Other items you might find at home:

- 2 tablespoon Hershey's Sugar Free Chocolate Syrup
- 4 ounces of V-8 Splash Piña Colada. This is great for Breakfast. Any V-8 drink goes good with our Egg Whites.
- 4 ounces Sunny-D Smooth. This is more concentrated than orange juice. If you want to use orange juice, use a fifty-fifty split of Egg Whites and OJ. Otherwise, it will taste like watered down orange juice.
- Starbucks single serving bottles make great high protein cold coffee drinks. Use 4 ounces to 6 ounces of any flavor coffee, with 8 ounces of Egg Whites, shake well.

You can take any coffee you like, add ice cubes for cold coffee, and add egg whites for a high protein breakfast and coffee combo (not hot coffee unless you want poached egg coffee).

# GOT KIDS WITH BAD EATING HABITS?

Can't get them to eat enough protein? Here's a quick trick for picky eaters (adults included!).

1/2 cup Egg Whites International
1/2 cup milk (1% 2% or whole)
1 bowl cereal of your choice

1.  Mix together in seconds and enjoy!

Your picky eater won't have a clue they just had 13 grams of pure egg white protein plus the added benefits of the milk and cereal nutrition!

You can also take the same mix of Egg Whites and Milk and just add chocolate syrup for a glass of chocolate "milk" containing 13 grams of pure egg white protein. Adults can use 8 ounces of Liquid Egg Whites for 26 grams of protein!

### FRUIT SMOOTHIE

1/2 banana
3 to 4 strawberries or use 1 cup strawberry/banana nectar
1/2 cup Egg Whites
1 cup pineapple or apple juice
1 cup ice cubes

1. Place fruit and ice in blender first and mix for 60 to 90 seconds.
2. Add Egg Whites and mix for another 10 to 15 seconds.

For thicker smoothie, just add more ice. For your personal favorite smoothie, just use juice or fruits desired.

### YOGURT SMOOTHIE

1/3 cup of low or nonfat plain or flavored yogurt
1/4 cup of fresh or canned pineapple or peaches
1/2 cup Egg Whites

1. Place in blender and mix for 10 to 15 seconds.

### EGG WHITE POPPERS

1 plastic ice cube tray enough Egg Whites to fill tray nonstick cooking spray

1. Coat ice cube tray with cooking spray
2. Pour in egg whites and microwave on high for 4 minutes
3. Refrigerate for 1 hour

You can experiment by mixing a small amount of sugar-free powdered Cool Aid Mix for flavor.

These are very popular with bodybuilders who will take these to the gym in a plastic ziplock bag and pop them in their mouth while working out. This gives them that extra protein boost during their workout.

### *JELL-O POPPERS*

1 plastic ice cube tray
Jell-O Mix (flavor of your choice!)
enough Egg Whites to fill tray
nonstick cooking spray

1. Coat ice cube tray with cooking spray.
2. Stir egg whites and powdered Jell-O Mix together and pour into tray.
3. Refrigerate until Jell-O poppers have set.

Like Egg White Poppers, these are very popular with bodybuilders who will take these to the gym in a plastic zip lock bag and pop them in their mouth while working out. This gives them that extra protein boost during their workout. Also great for sports activities like snowboarding and skiing!

### *TEXAS WHITE OMELET*

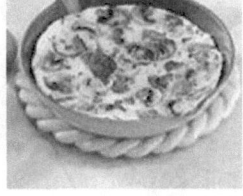

1 1/2 tablespoon olive or corn oil
1 cup Egg Whites
2 tablespoon chopped green/red peppers.
1 tablespoon chopped onion
1 tablespoon diced ham
1/4 cup grated cheddar cheese
Salt and Pepper to taste

1. Heat 1 tablespoon oil in a 9-inch nonstick frying pan.
2. Lightly sauté onions, peppers, and ham. Set aside.
3. Place 1/2 tablespoon of oil in pan at medium high heat.
4. Pour in Egg Whites.

As eggs begin to cook, lift sides to allow Egg Whites to set. While top of omelet is still moist, place the sautéed mixture on the omelet. Add Cheese if desired.

Using spatula, fold omelet in half. Be sure not to overcook. Season with salt and pepper as desired.

## *CALIFORNIA WHITE OMELET*

1 1/2 tablespoon olive or corn oil
1 cup Egg Whites
1 large mushroom (sliced up)
1 1/2 cup fresh spinach
1 tablespoon crumbled feta or goat cheese

1. Heat 1 tablespoon oil in a 9-inch frying pan.
2. Sauté spinach and mushrooms and then set aside.
3. Place 1/2 tablespoon oil into pan at medium high heat.
4. Pour in 1 cup Egg Whites.
5. As egg begins to cook, lift sides to allow Egg Whites to set.
6. While omelet is still moist, place spinach and mushrooms on top.
7. Sprinkle on cheese, fold omelet, and finish cooking.

## *BURRITO BAJA BREAKFAST*

4 8-inch fat free flour tortillas
3 tablespoon chopped green peppers
1/8 tablespoon salt, touch of pepper and cumin
1 cup Egg Whites
3 tablespoons diced tomato
1/4 cup shredded jalapeno cheese or cheddar
1 tablespoon olive or corn oil
1/2 cup of chorizo or diced meat of your choice

1. Place 1 tablespoon of oil in nonstick frying pan.
2. Season and cook green peppers for 2 min. (add meat if desired).
3. Add Egg Whites and scramble until fully cooked.
4. Stir in tomato.
5. Sprinkle 1/4 cup of cheese.
6. Spoon and roll in a tortilla.

# WHAT DOES IT REALLY TAKE?

How many times have you worked out, really worked your butt off for a period of time, and you get on the scale, and no change? Remember this, meaningful change takes place over a period of time. You will change, and you will transform your body, but you have to do it from the inside out! I truly believe that there are six rules of succeeding.

#1: ***Be Organized and Be Committed:*** To be successful you have to coordinate your time well, and you have to have a proper schedule. You will fail if you do not prepare and if you are not committed to the journey of your physical destination. Failing to Plan, is Planning to Fail.

#2: ***Write down your goals:*** I have always been a list writer, whether it is just things that I need to do on a certain day, or dreams, and goals. I firmly believe that when you write down your personal goals, you are more prone to staying on track. Start with short-term goals, mental and physical. Make a list of realistic goals that can be reached within a short amount of time. Then make a realistic list of long-term goals, ones that perhaps could be reached within eight to twelve months time. Whether you are just wanting to start with losing ten pounds, when you reach the goal, check it off and continue down the list. It is a wonderful way to keep your mental focus on your tasks at hand.

#3: ***Avoid temptations:*** No Excuses!. You must accomplish your objectives; otherwise, you have failed! COMMITMENT IS KEY. Do not let temptations get in the way of your goals and your accomplishments.

#4: ***Search for other success stories:*** Orientate yourself with other successful people. Surround yourself with others that have similar goals. Whenever you are doubtful about nutrition, training, supplements, or anything else always ask. Do your research. Find your motivation even if it is looking at fitness magazines or reading inspiring stories. Keep yourself in the moment for your own success story.

#5: *Combine:* A very important rule of thumb. Combine your workouts, should time cut you short. Think about it like this, it takes one missed workout to get you in a rut. Should you know that you are going to miss a workout, combine it with another, so you don't miss it. Make sure you prepare ahead of time for schedule changes so you don't falter back on the goals that you have already reached.

#6: **Be realistic:** You need to make sure that whatever your goals may be, you set realistic ones. Like I stated earlier, start small. There is no reason that you won't be able to reach whatever goals you may set, but be realistic with whatever you write down.

Bodybuilding and physical transformation, great or small, is complex. It involves every aspect of mind, body, and heart. They all must be in line and strong in order to succeed. Believe it when I say it is a mental game. You have to believe it in your mind and your heart to make it happen with your body. Keep your mind on track. Failing to plan is planning to fail. Determination makes a champion, no matter what your task, great or small. Make sure that your motivation is strong enough to get you where your goals are because if motivation is lost, all is lost. There is nothing more powerful than the power of prayer; I truly believe that in my heart. When you feel like you are losing your motivation, pray for mental and physical strength.

It has been a long journey for myself, and believe me when I say, the mental aspect of a complete transformation is one that comes and goes. I remember being invaded by Halloween candy and holiday goodies, but I made it through. My body does the same as everyone else's. I have ups and downs, good days and bad days. I give in to the little cravings, and then I suffer over it later, when I have to make up for an extra ten pounds that has found its way to my rear end. But ya know, I know what I have to do. I know that when I mess up and I give in, I need to put that mental focus back in my game. I don't know what the future holds, what competitions that I'll decide to get involved in, but I know that I won't be able to succeed at any of them if my mind and my heart is not in it. When I hear someone say, "I just don't have the time, the time to workout, or even mess with my diet," I hear that voice myself; and you know, I just make the time. When I look at my pictures before and several snapshots from over the years, I know in my heart that I don't ever want to be heavy again. I don't ever want to feel the way that I felt then—physically, emotionally, or mentally. I tell everyone that if I can do it, you can too. Don't let your mind become more of an obstacle than it should be. Take one day at a time. I had a lot of highs and lows over my transformation. I seem to put weight on just by looking at food or thinking about it. But I've come to the conclusion that I have to Eat to Live, not Live to Eat. There is a big difference, ya know. You can't let food overcome every aspect of your life. You have to have control over your decisions. Are they going make you or break you? Let your decisions make you who you want to be. Be strong, and you can accomplish anything that you put your heart, body, and mind to.

God bless you and Godspeed. May all your dreams, goals, and aspirations come true. Be true to yourself, and you will reap the benefits of a life and transformation fully accomplished. Then, and only then will you have honestly learned how to Eat to Live.

I want to thank Egg Whites International for a great life-changing product that helped me achieve my goals and enjoy doing it. Dieting was never so easy or tasted so good.

For more info on this great product, go to *www.eggwhitesint.com.* Or call 877-Egg-Whites.

To contact Kelli L. Harsha, please check out *www.phatchixfitness.com,* or e-mail at *phatchixfitness@yahoo.com*

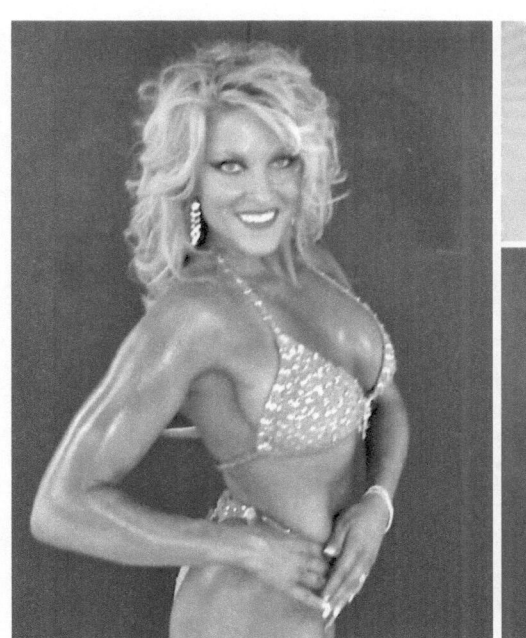
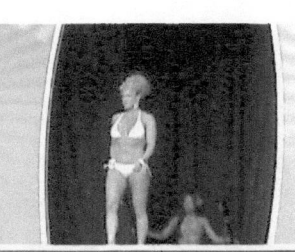
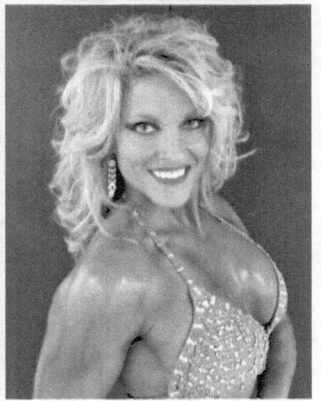
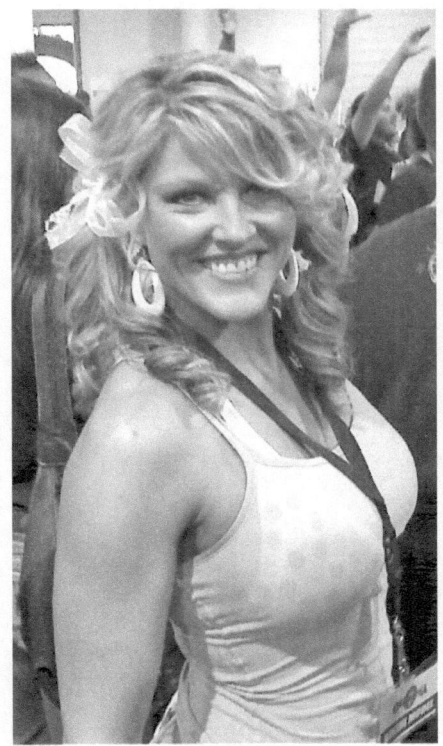
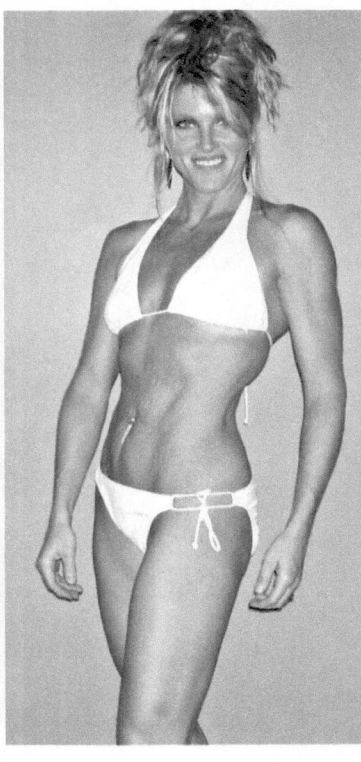